how to

Perform
Clinical
Procedures

how to Perform Clinical Procedures

Matthew Stephenson
Consultant General and Oncoplastic
Breast Surgeon
Jersey General Hospital

Joshua Shur
Foundation Trainee
South Thames Foundation School

John Black
Core Surgical Trainee
London Deanery

WILEY Blackwell

This edition first published 2013 © 2013 by John Wiley & Sons, Ltd

Registered Office
John Wiley & Sons, Ltd, The Atrium, Southern Gate, Chichester, West Sussex, PO19 8SQ, UK

Editorial Offices
9600 Garsington Road, Oxford, OX4 2DQ, UK
The Atrium, Southern Gate, Chichester, West Sussex, PO19 8SQ, UK
111 River Street, Hoboken, NJ 07030-5774, USA

For details of our global editorial offices, for customer services and for information about how
to apply for permission to reuse the copyright material in this book please see our website at
www.wiley.com/wiley-blackwell

Library of Congress Cataloging-in-Publication Data

Stephenson, Matthew, author.
How to perform clinical procedures / Matthew Stephenson, Joshua Shur, John Black.
    p. ; cm.
  Includes bibliographical references and index.
  ISBN 978-0-470-65858-1 (paperback : alk. paper)
I. Shur, Joshua, author.   II. Black, John, 1985- author.   III. Title.
[DNLM: 1. Surgical Procedures, Operative.   2. Clinical Competence.   3. Clinical Medicine–methods.
WO 500]
  RD37
  617–dc23
                                        2013018955

A catalogue record for this book is available from the British Library.

Wiley also publishes its books in a variety of electronic formats. Some content that appears in print may
not be available in electronic books.

Cover images: Courtesy of the authors
Cover design by Daniel R. James

Set in 8.5/12pt Helvetica by SPi Publisher Services, Pondicherry, India
Printed and bound in Singapore by Markono Print Media Pte Ltd

1 2013

Acknowledgements

The authors would like to thank the following who have either been filmed or who have helped review a chapter:

Vivienne Andrews (Bone Marrow Aspirate and Biopsy)

Saif Baluch (Ascitic Tap)

Mike Barrett (Local Anaesthetic Infiltration)

Antonia Benton (Ring Block)

Deborah Bolton (Arterial Blood Gas, Venepuncture-Peripheral, Intravenous Fluid Infusion, Intravenous Injection, Central Venous Line, Peripheral Venous Cannulation, Blood Cultures)

Nikesh Chandarana (Endotracheal Intubation)

Sue Dawson (Nasogastric Tube)

Uzma Faruqi (Large Bore Chest Drain Removal)

Ali Fawzi (Pleural Tap)

Andrew Fish (Gynaecological Examination and Cervical Smear)

Sally Goodman (Urinary Catheter-Female, Urinary Catheter-Male)

Patience Gosha (Blood Transfusion)

Richard Harvey (Suturing)

Amanda Heitmann (Pleural Aspiration)

Minija Joseph (Urinary Catheter-Female)

Norman Kock (Lumbar Puncture)

Michael Lincoln (Observations, Capillary Blood Glucose)

Emma Lyall (Spirometry)

Michael Marrinan (Large Bore Chest Drain Removal)

Caroline Martin (Intravenous Injection)

Julie Millest (Peak Flow)

Hiren Mistry (Suturing)

Beata Misztal (Cardioversion)

Clare Morley (Electrocardiogram)

Mungo Morris (Flexible Nasendoscopy)

Lana Nela (Cardioversion)

Therese Phelan (Intramuscular Injection)

Mark Prince (Peak Flow)

Tajwinder Sandhar (Nasogastric Tube)

Lynne Schofield (Venesection)

Nabil Siddique (Lumbar Puncture)

Helen Slator (Intravenous Fluid Infusion)

Sonia Vanner (Nebuliser)

Yvonne Wesley (Scrubbing)

Rupert Williams (Cardioversion)

With particular thanks for their filming contributions:

Dr Liam Mahoney, BMBS, MRCPCH
ST 2 Paediatrics & Honorary Teaching Fellow
Brighton & Sussex University Hospitals NHS Trust

Dr Patrick Thorburn, MBChB, BSc (Hons)
Anaesthetic Trainee

And especially, for his film editing and producing:

Mr Daniel James

We also thank the following for their help: Ginny Bowbrick; Jonathan Compson; Philip Dart; Catherine Fularton; Aisling Hillary; David Hutchinson; Liz Green; Ruochen Li; Eric Lindberg; Caroline Martin; Logini Saivanathan; Rizwan Saleem; Geoffrey Warwick; Jamie Weber-Macartney.

Personal acknowledgements

Josh: Thanks to my parents Rose and Eric and to my sister Nat, for all their advice and wisdom. Thanks to Matt, John and Dan with their never-ending patience. Last but not least thanks of course to Phi-Anh for supporting me the whole way.

John: I would like to thank:

- Lois Black, a truly remarkable mother and absolute one in a million – apart from being my maker and my best friend, you always said that what I didn't know, I'd put down in a book one day – so here you are!
- The marvellous healthcare professionals involved in making this project possible – a pleasure to work with you all.
- And finally … my co-authors, Matthew and Joshua – I'm so glad you agreed on *all* my suggestions – *all* of the time.'

Contents

List of Contributors

Primary authors

Matthew Stephenson, MBBS, BSc, MSc, FRCS (gen surg)
Consultant General and Oncoplastic
Breast Surgeon
Jersey General Hospital

Joshua Shur, MBBS, MSci (Hons)
Foundation Trainee
South Thames Foundation School

John Black, BMBS, BA (Hons) Music
Core Surgical Trainee
London Deanery

Contributors

Dr Stephanie Ball, BMBS
Core Medical Trainee (Gastroenterology)
Queens Medical Centre, Nottingham
*Appendix 3 – How To Be an Even
Better F2*

Dr Adrian Barnardo, BMedSci(Hons), BM, BS, MD, MRCP
Consultant Gastroenterologist
Medway Maritime Hospital, Gillingham
Ascitic Tap
Ascitic Drain

Mr Michael Barrett, MBChb, MRCS
Core Surgical Trainee (Plastic Surgery)
Queen Victoria Hospital, East Grinstead
Local Anaesthetic Infiltration

Mrs Angeline Boorer
Infection Control Nurse
Royal Sussex County Hospital,
Brighton
Hand Hygiene

Dr Rosemary Chester, BMBS
Foundation Year 2 Doctor
Maidstone Hospital,
Maidstone
Subcutaneous Injection
*Appendix 2 – How To
Be a Great F1*

Ms Joy Edlin, MRCS
Core Surgical Trainee
Hillingdon Hospital, Uxbridge
Large Bore Chest Drain
Seldinger Chest Drain

Dr Sarah Fisher, MBChb
Foundation Year 1 Doctor
King's College Hospital
London Deanery
Upper Limb Backslab

Dr Vanessa Fludder, MBBS, FRCA, PGCME
Consultant Anaesthetist
Brighton and Sussex University
Hospitals
Spinal Injection

Mr Bertram Fu, MBChB, DO-HNS, MRCSEd
Specialty Registrar in Otolaryngology
London Deanery
Flexible Nasendoscopy

Mr Alan Giles
Senior Orthopaedic Technician
King's College Hospital,
London
Upper Limb Backslab

Dr John Gomes, MA, MBBS, MRCP
Cardiology Registrar
Royal Sussex County Hospital,
Brighton
Cardioversion

Mr George Goumalatsos, Ptychio Iatrikes, MRCOG
ST6 in Obstetrics and Gynaecology
London/KSS Deanery
Gynaecological Exam and Cervical Smear

Miss Shelly Griffiths, MBBS, MA (Cantab), MRCS
Core Surgical Trainee
Peninsula Deanery
Surgical Scubbing

Mr Meredydd Harries, FRCS, MSc
Consultant ENT & Voice Surgeon
Royal Sussex County Hospital,
Brighton
Flexible Nasendoscopy

Dr David Kirtchuk, MBBS
Foundation Year 2 Doctor
Medway Maritime Hospital, Gillingham
Urinary Catheter – Male

Mr Michael Marrinan, FRCS (Ed)
Consultant Thoracic Surgeon
Executive Medical Director
King's College Hospital, London
Large Bore Chest Drain
Seldinger Chest Drain

Dr Christopher Parnell, MB, FRCA
Lead Consultant for Vascular
Anaesthesia
Medway NHS Foundation Trust
Arterial Cannulation
Central Venous Line
Endotracheal Intubation
Epidural
Peripheral Venous Cannulation

Dr Elizabeth Ratcliffe, MBBS (Hons), BmedSci
Foundation Year 2 Doctor
Medway Maritime Hospital, Gillingham
Urinary Catheter – Male

Dr Anita Sarma, MBChb, BSc
Specialist Registrar, Haematology
King's College Hospital, London Deanery
Bone Marrow Biopsy and Aspirate

Dr Charlotte Smith, MBBS, BSc (Hons)
ST3 in Obstetrics & Gynaecology
London/KSS Deanery
Gynaecological Exam and Cervical Smear

Dr Emma Stewart-Parker, BM, MA(Cantab)
Core Surgical Trainee
Kings College Hospital, London Deanery
Intramuscular Injection

Mr Stuart John Wind, AVS, MSc (KCL & Exon)
Vascular Sonographer
North Shore Vascular Laboratory
NSW, Australia
Ankle Brachial Pressure Index

Dr Reshma Woograsingh, BSc, MBBS, FRCA
Senior Specialty Registrar in Anaesthetics
North Central Thames School of Anaesthesia
Arterial Cannulation
Central Venous Line
Endotracheal Intubation
Epidural

Dr Arthee Yogendran, MBBS, BA (Hons), MA (Cantab)
Foundation Year 2 Doctor
Medway Maritime Hospital, Gillingham
Arterial Blood Gas

Foreword

This is a brilliant practical book and DVDs of basic clinical procedures written chiefly by medical and surgical doctors in training with contributions from more experienced clinicians. Like all good books I wonder why it had not been thought of before. It covers a large range of procedures from handwashing to central venous cannulation and has excellent text for each with useful text boxes and OSCE type checklists, and then a simple video with commentary. Being written by those who have to do these daily by trainees, it is eminently sensible and practical, and it reminds its readers of things that are easily forgotten. In some areas there is useful medical information. There are three excellent appendices on obtaining consent, being a good and better junior trainee, and applying for jobs. I only wish it had been available a while ago!

Safety and quality are now essential, and every patient wants a competent procedure. No longer can these procedures be done without practice or at least simulation training. This publication will add to such preparation and I am sure will be welcomed by its audience. I wish it well and hope that all deaneries, postgraduate centres and trainers will encourage its use.

Sir Richard Thompson, KCVO, DM, PRCP
President
Royal College of Physicians

Preface

When you hit the age of 17 in the United Kingdom, or 16 in the United States, statistically your chances of killing someone increases dramatically. Why? Because the first thing on your mind is to get a driving licence. And there's a reason why motor insurance is so pricey for new young drivers. If you're a medical student or junior doctor reading this book one of the most exciting things to learn as early as possible is clinical procedures. It starts off with taking venous blood, moves on to intravenous cannulae and, if you're lucky (and work hard), it won't be long before you're putting in chest drains and suturing wounds.

When you're starting off in medicine, doing these procedures brings great personal reward – doing a cardioversion is much more fun than reading about the Krebs cycle. But just like driving, it also marks the beginning of a time in which you can potentially cause harm to real people. That's what this book is about – teaching you to understand the procedure and how to perform it properly.

Taking the driving analogy a bit further, in the driving test, before manoeuvring you need to make an obvious show of turning your head to check the mirror for example. Many of the undergraduate (and some postgraduate) exams are a bit like this, especially those that are in an Objective Structured Clinical Examination (OSCE) format. You will enter the examination room and the examiner will have a very specific checklist he/she will go through – and to score all the points you must demonstrate all of the points on the list. In real life, in the rough and tumble of working on busy hospital wards and when you've been doing these procedures for years, many clinicians 'fine tune' how they do their procedure. Usually this is due to time constraint reasons. Sometimes this equates to 'falling into bad habits', but often it's just pragmatic reasoned streamlining; however, when you learn procedures for the first time you want to learn the 'right' way of doing them. If you realise later in your career that doing something differently, but still safely, works for you then so be it. But learning the mainstream, commonly accepted approach is the right way to start out. The problem though is that there is no bible of procedure techniques, there is no comprehensive, internationally agreed resource. If you took 10 anaesthetists, they would all show you a slightly different way of putting a venflon in. This variability is reflected in the fact that there is no standard OSCE marksheet. These vary by medical school or postgraduate examining board. Furthermore, trends change over time and certain techniques go in and out of fashion. Using the trocar in a chest drain went out the window years ago. Then ultrasound became mandatory as part of putting in central lines. More recently doctors have been banned from wearing white coats in clinical areas. A clinical procedures video like this from 20 years ago (were one to have been in existence) would look very different. Forty years ago it wouldn't be surprising if the doctor was puffing away on a cigarette whilst he jiggled the lumbar puncture into the subarachnoid space with his ungloved hand. Times change and one wonders what the next generation will say about how we do things now.

So how have we tried to cope with this lack of consistency? You will find in this book and DVDs a wide range of procedures, from diagnostic to treatment, non-invasive to invasive. We have tried to film each procedure being done in *an* acceptable way, not necessarily *the* way that it's done in your hospital, but a way which would be entirely acceptable to any body of medical practitioners.

For some procedures there are in fact national guidelines in place, for instance for chest drains, and where this is the case we have incorporated these into the video and discussed them in the book. If there are other particular issues of controversy or debate, we've tried to pay lip service to these too. In all cases, the video and chapter has been reviewed by either a consultant, senior nurse or technician, depending on the appropriateness of the procedure.

So this lack of consistency is all reflected in the OSCE marksheets. These have been carefully constructed having assessed and cross referenced numerous OSCE marksheets from various institutions. As a result they are comprehensive – and often contain more checklist points than you would expect in the average OSCE, so don't lost heart if some of them seem dauntingly long.

'I'm never going to get a cardioversion in my OSCE,' I hear you say. Probably not. However many of the procedures are eminently examinable by OSCE and frequently are included in exams, such as peripheral intravenous cannulation. So to maintain consistency, we've used the same OSCE checklist style for *all* the videos, even if only to double as a clear summary of the steps. It's worth remembering though, that OSCE style exams have increased, and continue to increase in popularity – don't be too surprised if one of the more esoteric ones comes up.

But life isn't all about exams: providing first class clinical care to your patients is infinitely more important than what you can demonstrate with a urinary catheter on a plastic model to a half-asleep examiner. However ultimately, the idea of this book and DVDs is that it will equip you with the knowledge and understanding to both approach performing procedures yourself on real patients, but also to pass your OSCEs.

There are some procedures here that doubtless you'll be shaking your head and thinking 'but that's the nurses job!'

It's true that the nurse's role has changed dramatically over the last 20 years. If you were an F1 in the 1980s you'd have been doing every blood test, every cannula *and* preparing and giving all the intravenous medications! However all of these are still core skills, and there's no excuse not to know how to take a patient's "obs" or dip their urine. You can't always rely on a nurse to be free to help you.

Learning to perform clinical procedures has never been so tough. The European Working Time Directive has reduced the amount of time you spend in the hospital seeing patients. It has also had a knock on effect on training time versus service time, with more time spent on nights where non-urgent procedures will be deferred until the morning. There may also be more doctors added to your rota, meaning more competition for experience. You want to get yourself to a high enough standard as quickly as possible so that if there's a lumbar puncture or a cardioversion happening you get to do it, within reason, as early in your career as you can. There are a variety of *training-the-trainers* type courses. One of the educational mantras is a four-stage teaching technique essentially breaking down the advice to the trainer as:

1 Perform the procedure at a normal pace with the trainee watching without explanation, as you would normally do it.
2 Perform the procedure at a pace to allow the trainee to see and understand each step with explanations as you go.

3 Perform the procedure but have the trainee tell you what to do next.
4 Let the trainee perform the procedure explaining all the steps to you.

So if you've at least watched the procedure, maybe a handful of times from one of these videos, the first time you see it in vivo it won't be so unfamiliar, getting you a leg up on the learning curve that little bit earlier. In fact potentially straight on to stage 3 or 4. Clearly nobody, hopefully, is going to stick rigidly to that mantra – otherwise it would mean if you have been in a six-month job and only three ascitic drains have come up (when you're not on nights / annual leave / study leave / post nights enforced compensatory rest / pre night's enforced compensatory rest / covering someone else / on call) by these rules you wouldn't have even got your hands on one of them, so it of course needs adaptability from the trainer. But your trainer is likely to be substantially more adaptable if you come to work preloaded with the knowledge. *Proper Prior Planning Prevents Piss Poor Performance* as they say.

You might be interested to know that there are four stages of competence:

1 **Unconscious incompetence**: You really haven't the first idea how much you don't know/can't do.
2 **Conscious incompetence**: You begin to realise how little you know / can do, and can't do it.
3 **Conscious competence**: Suddenly, you know stuff / can do stuff and you know it.

4 Unconscious competence: Gradually, without you noticing, you know stuff / can do stuff but you've known it for so long the novelty's worn off and it's second nature (this is often the reason for the phenomenon of the pant wetting stage of 'I don't know *anything*' just before an exam, followed by acing it).

Hopefully this book and DVD will catapult you out of any stage 1-ishness you have about you into stage 2, and combined with actually performing the procedures, direct you into that wondrous, life-assuring, endorphin-releasing stage 3 – you can put in a chest drain, and you know it.

Making this DVD

We are a high definition, surround sound, 3D, watch-on-demand, interactive-press-the-red-button generation. We demand a lot from what we watch, and we are used to certain standards when it comes to watching videos or TV. Those standards are set by professional cameramen and professional directors in professional editing suites. We are doctors. We have tried our very, very best to get the right shots of the right things for you. However, we are just jobbing medics, with limited videographic expertise. For that reason, whilst we're very proud of the videos, they're probably not the same as you'd get from a professional camera crew. But we realised early on in the process that wasn't practical for all sorts of logistical reasons: patients don't want to be intimidated by a film crew when they're having an intimate moment with a needle. And when

procedures happen is unpredictable so we'd need to have a film crew on standby 24/7 (in which case you'd have paid a lot more for this product).

In the first book in this *How to* series, *How to Operate*, I learnt how difficult it is to do a video project like this. You really can't imagine. For some time I was amazed at why no one else had tried it before on this scale, it gradually became clear why no one has. First there was the clearance from the legal departments of the Trusts (more than one to increase the yield), ensure all the right paperwork was in order, from cycling proficiency test certificates to hepatitis B immunisations. Then to find the right pathology, in the right patient, who consented to being filmed (actually the easiest thing in the process, we owe our patients a huge amount, our patients were often the most enthusiastic people in the whole project), with the right doctor or nurse at the right time in the right place, with the right person and equipment (which works) available to film it: tricky. Some procedures are easier to film than others for obvious reasons. So you may be thinking *why on earth have they included procedure A and not B?* Yes we agree – we would have loved to include every procedure that you might ever encounter. This, however, would have taken a very, very, very long time. We have tried to get *the* essential procedures, with a few special ones thrown in. For the aforementioned reasons, it's simply not possible to get everything on film, so please forgive us, but we have tried.

Generic Principles in Clinical Procedures

There are several common themes and principles in performing clinical procedures and it would be tedious to keep repeating them in each chapter. So here's a ragbag of thoughts, topics and issues to think about, in no particular order.

Primum non nocere.
First, do no harm

Many procedures, especially invasive ones, come with risks. It sounds obvious, but don't do a procedure if you don't have to. If you've been asked by a nurse to go and put in a cannula for a patient's antibiotics, spare a moment to think: does the patient really need intravenous antibiotics? Could they be switched to orals saving the patient the pain of the cannulation and the infection risks? Maybe not, but just consider it.

Within this category you need also to make sure that you are operating within the boundaries of your competencies. If you're asked by a senior to go and put a chest drain in and you've never done one –

you must say. If you're coerced into performing procedures you feel are beyond your competencies, you must stand up for yourself, and the patient – *patient safety* comes first. This dovetails into the next issue.

Ask for help

If you're unsure, ask for help. Simple. Foundation doctors should now have substantial protection and supervision, the days of being left alone to do all sorts of complex invasive procedures on your first day should be well and truly over. There is no shame in asking for help. If you're going to be doing a procedure you're competent to do alone but still haven't done that many, make sure you have the number to hand of your senior and that they're available if things go awry.

Be humane

Patients are people. A certain air of detachment from this can be helpful in some contexts, particularly in surgery; for instance when you have your hands deep in someone's abdomen it's usually more productive to consider the biological machine you have in front of you, rather than the person you've been talking to. It's this emotional detachment that allows doctors to do some of the pretty peculiar things we do to patients. But allowing this to go too far is a common problem. Talk to patients, tell them what you're going to do and be sure that they understand and agree to it. Be kind, warn them if you're about to cause them pain, and there's a gentleness in saying sorry for it even if it's necessary. Don't expose patients unnecessarily, especially for intimate procedures like urinary catheters. For instance set up all your equipment and be sure you're ready, and then uncover the patient, covering them back up again afterwards as soon as possible. Respect people's dignity.

Don't get disheartened

We all have bad days. If you're struggling to get to grips with a procedure, you're not alone. Intravenous cannulae are the commonest procedure for people to struggle with early on. A patient with big superficial veins is easy to cannulate, but when you've had five patients on the trot all with no veins to speak of, you tend to get downhearted. All we can say is: we've all been there. Try not to let the bad experience of the last one affect the next one you do, or the negative vibes will rub off on your chances of subsequent success. The phenomenon of losing your cannula 'mojo' is common – everyone will experience it, so don't get disheartened. The only answer to struggling with procedures is (a) make sure you've got the technique right (have a senior watch you do it) and (b) do loads of them. This means that if your patient needs a cannula, or whatever, even if a nurse very kindly offers to do it – do it yourself! By the end of your first F1 rotation you should be able to cannulate the 'worst' of arms and the only way to get that good is to have done hundreds of them. It may seem like a bonus that the nurses on your ward can cannulate (and sometimes it is when you're super busy), but don't make the mistake of not getting skilled yourself.

Instill confidence

You will of course develop your own natural way of interacting with patients – it's a highly personal thing. However within it you have to learn how to make your patient reassured that they are in safe hands. Sometimes this can be very hard to do when your own sweaty palms risk giving you away. Instilling confidence doesn't simply mean telling the patient everything's going to be OK (especially considering that sometimes it's not, that's the whole point of telling patients about potential complications, although you can help them to retain a balance on this), it means looking the part, and sometimes you have to do a bit of acting. Obviously this doesn't mean winging it – if you are nervous because you're not actually competent to do the procedure – you shouldn't be doing it. But if you're looking anxious simply because you're still relatively new, this is what you must learn to hide from your patient. Unfortunately, this attempt at hiding your nerves often doesn't have the intended result. Some of the most arrogant, pompous and condescending doctors are doing exactly this – trying to disguise their own anxieties – but it ends up making them look like a prat. You just have to learn a way that's natural for you to look confident and self-assured – that's what your patient wants.

Document it

If it's not written down, it didn't happen. You will hear this repeated *ad nauseam*, but there's truth to it. If it's not documented there's no evidence it happened. If you're involved in a complaint or even litigation months or even years down the line, there is absolutely no chance you will remember anything about the procedure, you will only be able to rely on what you wrote down at the time. Regardless, documenting things is the only reliable way of communicating what happened to the other people looking after that patient. This point is so important we cannot really overstate it.

Follow local protocol

Every hospital is different and this can manifest in some minor or major differences in how some procedures should be done. Be sure to familiarise yourself as early as possible with the policies, protocols and guidelines of that trust. These have almost invariably been written because something bad has happened in the past and they don't want the mistake to be repeated. Often they seem daft. Obey them anyway. Protocols should be adhered to strictly unless there is strong reason not to. Why? Because if you go against hospital protocol and something goes wrong your hospital (or strictly speaking the NHS Litigation Authority) will more than likely not back you up and you'll be relying on your own medical defence/protection company. Guidelines are a looser affair, offering you a sensible way of doing something, which in general should be followed. Policies, protocols and guidelines are almost always available on the hospital's Intranet. It may seem like the most boring thing in the world to do on your first week of being an F1 but it's worth setting aside an evening to read all the ones that you think might be relevant to you.

Get consent

To avoid repetition just read Appendix 1 for full details.

Procedures

Cleanliness

Hand hygiene

If there's one thing that's guaranteed to bug a doctor, it's telling them how to wash their hands. This simple task is now even part of most hospital inductions. You know how to wash your hands for goodness sake, don't you? You've been doing it since you were three! Well, that may be, but actually trusts are right to labour the point because it's surprising how many doctors don't wash their hands properly. If you haven't yet been subjected to an ultraviolet light test to check the effectiveness of your hand-washing, this particular joy awaits you, sometimes as a complete surprise by the infection control nurse on the ward, sometimes in front of a large lecture audience. If there's one thing in the whole infection control debate for which there is strong evidence, it's washing your hands. For this reason, we've devoted an entire chapter to hand hygiene, so for more on the seven-stage technique, alcohol gels and other joys, read ahead! Having read that chapter you will become very familiar with the 'five moments for hand hygiene'; you will also hopefully then understand why we don't in the chapters constantly go on about washing your hands in between each step of the procedure – it would become very tedious. You need to use your common sense, and this 'five moments' business to guide you when you need to wash your hands, in addition to the obvious beginning and end of each procedure.

Follow infection control guidelines

Because of the relatively recent rise in, and publicity around, hospital-acquired infections, infection control is now a big deal in the NHS. There is a lot of bad blood between the infection control 'police' and doctors, especially senior ones. This generally is because of the flimsy, or in some cases non-existent, evidence base for some of these policies. Many doctors believe that in fact these are a smokescreen for the real problems that cause infection outbreaks, such as maximal bed occupancy resulting in inadequate time for cleaning and excessive opportunities for interpatient contact, etc. We could not possibly comment, our only advice would be: Follow infection control policies! If your ageing consultant wants to start a war with the infection control team by not rolling up his sleeves, let him do it. You as a junior haven't a leg to stand on and will only make trouble for yourself. So in general, and without comment on the validity of these:

- Bare below the elbows! Sleeves should be rolled up to above the elbow, this means that jackets etc. are removed at the door.
- Wrist watches must not be worn (most people attach them to their belt instead).
- Ties are banned in many trusts; others let you wear them if they're tucked in.
- Most trusts will have specific rules about jewellery, many limiting you to just a wedding ring.
- Don't have the lanyard round your neck with your ID card in it flopping around in front of you when you're doing a procedure; you don't want it dangling into bodily fluids.
- There is usually a ban on white coats in clinical areas.

- There are many more depending on the trust – find out what they are, and follow the letter of the law.

Personal protective equipment

For procedures involving bodily fluids, you must wear gloves. In some procedures, such as taking blood, these can be non-sterile but for aseptic and sterile procedures (see individual chapters) they must be sterile. Be aware of latex allergies and be sure to avoid using latex gloves anywhere near a latex allergic patient. You should also wear a plastic disposable apron for any procedure involving bodily fluids. For patients known to be at high infection risk (e.g. Hepatitis C or HIV) take extra precautions – double glove and wear an eye visor as a minimum. The so-called *universal* precautions, are named as such simply because they must be applied *universally*, you are assuming all patients are an equal infection risk. You should stick to these rigorously.

However with all these precautions the most important thing is to simply be careful. In addition some people find double gloves can increase clumsiness.

For sterile procedures there is a scale from sterile gloves and a non-sterile apron to full surgical attire, that is, a face mask with an eye visor, hat, a full surgical scrub, followed by donning a sterile gown and sterile gloves (see Chapter 36: Surgical Scrubbing). See the individual chapters for which is most appropriate.

Non-sterile gloves come in small, medium and large. Sterile gloves can too, but more often they come in glove sizes. These range from tiny (5.5) to massive (9) in 0.5 increments. The average for a woman is 6.5–7 and for a man, 7–7.5.

Sharps

Dispose of your sharps *immediately* after you have used them. This usually means taking a portable sharps bin to the patient's bedside (although some trusts prefer to have fewer, large sharps bins in designated areas; as we have said before, check your trust's guidelines). Never resheath a needle. Of course 99 times out of 100 you'd do it safely, but when you're tired at the end of a long shift, if that's the habit you've got into, you're setting yourself up for a stab. Never overfill a sharps bin. *Never* reach in to a sharps bin to retrieve something you accidentally put in there.

If you do inadvertently sustain a sharps injury immediately vigorously wash the puncture site in running water and soap and try to squeeze out blood. Follow your hospital's protocol on sharps injuries which usually involves during daylight hours visiting the occupational health department and out of hours, the Emergency Department. The patient may need to be consented for hepatitis and HIV status if it is not known. Take sharps injuries seriously – don't just pretend it didn't happen, act on it and learn from it.

Clean vs aseptic vs sterile procedures

What do we mean by **clean**? Pretty much everything you do at work should be clean – it means the sensible precautions you take in washing your hands at every opportunity and not sneezing in patient's wounds. It's the steps you take before examining patients or taking blood for instance.

Aseptic means the absence of resident microorganisms and requires a good hand-wash followed by drying them with non-sterile towels, sterile gloves and anti-septic on the skin, as a minimum. This is for some invasive procedures such as insertion of a urinary catheter.

Sterile means the absence of all microorganisms and is reserved for the most invasive procedures, particularly where there is a risk of bacteraemia. Many of the procedures in this book fit this description, such as central venous line insertion and epidural. This requires:

- a hat
- a mask – more for your own protection
- eye protection
- a full surgical scrub
- hands dried with sterile towels
- sterile theatre gown

- sterile gloves
- sterile skin prep
- sterile drapes to create a sterile field
- all sterile equipment opened in a sterile fashion onto a sterile field
- ideally a dedicated clean room (e.g. theatre) although not always possible especially in an emergency

With aseptic and sterile techniques you need to get used to the concept of your clean area. This is usually set up on a portable table/trolley which you must first wipe down (you don't know where it's been) with an alcohol wipe. You need to lay a water impermeable sterile drape over this and then open all of your sterile equipment on to it. In practice, this sterile drape is usually simply created by opening up a 'sterile pack' – the inner surface of the outer layer of the sterile pack becomes the drape. Next to this you should open up your yellow clinical waste bag (which comes in your sterile pack) and if sharps are involved, have your sharps bin next to it. The **sterile pack**, by the way, is a ubiquitous product

	Clean	Aseptic	Sterile
Where?	Bedside/clinic	Bedside but ideally dedicated room	Ideally dedicated clean room
Gloves	Non-sterile or none if non-invasive	Sterile	Sterile
Hand hygiene	Routine	Hand washing or alcohol gel	Surgical scrub
Hand drying	Routine	Non-sterile towels	Sterile towels
Skin cleaning	Alcohol wipe if invasive	Long acting skin prep, e.g. chlorhexidine or iodine	Long acting skin prep, e.g. chlorhexidine or iodine
Sterile field	No	Sometimes	Always
Sterile gown	No	Not usually	Yes

throughout NHS hospitals and usually contains: some sterile gauze, a pot (to put your cleaning solution in), some plastic forceps, a paper sterile drape and of course the very useful outer layer mentioned above.

Remember that there should be a 'work flow' through your sterile area. For instance, your assistant drops some sterile gauze into your sterile work space and pours some cleaning solution into your pot, also in the sterile work space. You then clean the patient's skin with said skin-prep soaked gauze – you don't then return it to your sterile workspace, you must consider it dirty and it goes straight into the yellow clinical waste bag. Once you have made the area of the patient clean too you can then return your equipment to the sterile tray once it's been used on the patient, however if you inadvertently touch something that's not been cleaned – do not return it to your sterile area!

Cleaning the skin

There are three main types of skin prep based on iodine, povidone-iodine and ethyl alcohol. Each has its own advantages and disadvantages – your hospital may have a preference for which you use, find out. Ideally the skin should be cleaned by a swab, 'remotely', that is, you hold the swab using a pair of forceps so that your gloves don't risk coming into contact with as yet unclean skin, if you don't have this luxury, just take care not to touch the skin as you do it. Clean the skin starting in the middle, that is, where your procedure is about to take place, and then work out spirally in circles. Repeat this once. Give the skin prep time to work before diving in, especially with alcohol based cleaning solutions which must be allowed time to dry.

Whether to use local for quick procedures

There is debate over whether to use local anaesthetic for procedures that last almost only as long as it takes to put the local in, for instance arterial cannulation. Those that don't do it say that it's not helpful because the pain of the local is as bad as the procedure and it wastes times and resources. Also it causes a swelling under the skin, making it more difficult to palpate what you're feeling for.

Advocates for using local say that actually if the procedure does take longer than you were expecting (e.g. if you don't get the needle in first time) at least the area is numb whilst you have another go, and another go. One strong argument for using local is that whilst local is painful to put in, the pain wears off in a few seconds and the area goes completely numb. Without local, the patient can still feel the pain of a big needle inserted (into the radial artery for instance) for many minutes to come.

In short, it's up to you and your patient. A middle ground is the use of topical anaesthetic agents which work variably and take a while to take effect – certainly these are best for children.

Some quick miscellaneous things

- **Get everything set up in advance**: It's difficult to go back for things when you've put your sterile gloves on especially if you have no assistant. Take a spare of everything you think you might fail to get in the first time.
- **French and Gauge**: The diameter of needles, catheters etc. are usually described in either French scale or Gauge. 1 French equates to a diameter of 1/3 mm, for example, 12F = 4 mm. Gauge is usually used for needles, and confusingly the smaller the number, the larger the needle. You don't need to know the millimetres the Gauge refers to but suffice to say that the main ones in use are:

  21G – Green – commonly used for taking blood for instance;

  23G – Blue – commonly used for instilling local anaesthetic for instance;

  25G – Orange – commonly used for instilling local anaesthetic for instance.

- **Practice on models**: If you have the opportunity, practise your techniques on specially made simulators. For some procedures, such as interrupted suturing, ask to borrow the equipment from theatre and practice on an orange or banana.
- **National guidance**: Keep an eye out on the National Patient Safety Agency (NPSA) and National Institute for Clinical Evidence (NICE) websites for updates on guidance for procedures.

Finally, we would just like to say: good luck! Getting stuck in and involved with practical procedures can be daunting, frustrating yet immensely satisfying. We hope this resource will help you.

1 Ankle Brachial Pressure Index

Stuart Wind

Video Time | 3 mins 42 s

Overview

The **Ankle-Brachial Pressure Index** (ABPI) is a very useful non-invasive test which can quickly identify the presence and severity of peripheral arterial disease. As a result it's widely used by clinicians, and whilst different hospitals have different teams responsible for doing the test itself, such as vascular scientists or vascular nurses, at some point the task of performing an ABPI will fall to you. The other advantage with this test over some of the others mentioned in this book is that you can practise on a colleague. This is helpful as it frequently pops up in OSCEs. Performing it is easy; being able to look slick and perform the test accurately and reproducibly is another matter; this requires a little practice.

Don't worry, the ABPI is a very simple test and can be fun to perform, since it often brings not only a sense of relief, but often some amusement for the patient who, upon hearing the amplified signal from the handheld Doppler, will realise that they are in fact alive with a strange sound in their leg. Nevertheless there are a number of pitfalls which you can fall into for instance with inverted champagne bottle shaped and oedematous painful legs, so please read on carefully.

Procedure

Make sure you have the **correct patient**, for the **correct procedure**. Check for any **allergies** (unlikely to be an issue in this procedure), and that you have confirmed the **indication;** excluded any **contraindications; explained** the procedure and taken **consent**. Now **wash your hands**!

Assemble all of your equipment on a trolley away from the patient. You will need everything in the equipment textbox. Make sure that you have the **appropriate**

How to Perform Clinical Procedures, First Edition. Matthew Stephenson, Joshua Shur and John Black.
© 2013 John Wiley & Sons, Ltd. Published 2013 by John Wiley & Sons, Ltd.

Indications	Contraindications	Complications
• Screening for or grading peripheral arterial disease • Determining if the patient is suitable for compression bandaging (e.g. in chronic venous insufficiency) • Ruling out arterial contribution to ulceration • Assessing degree of success of revascularisation procedures	• Patients with excessive lower limb pain (e.g. reflex sympathetic dystrophy, severe circumferential ulceration, cellulitis) (relative) • Recent (<6 months) DVT (relative)	• Nil significant

kit for your patient, for example correct-sized blood pressure cuff. If the patient has any open wounds or ulcers you can cover these with **dressings or sterile cling film** as the test can be inaccurate if performed over bandaging. Emphasising the importance of **lying flat** should increase compliance in patients who have trouble being supine for long due to heart failure for instance. Being flat will avoid errors due to changes in blood pressure introduced by posture. There are few patients who can't lie flat for just a few moments but those who can't can have an extra pillow or the head end of the couch raised slightly. Furthermore, especially for the occasions when a patient has walked from afar to see you, make sure that they have **rested for at least 10 minutes** before commencing the test so that systolic blood pressure stabilises.

Firstly you should **take the brachial systolic pressure** as this will give you

an idea of what to expect at the ankle. The systolic pressure is the only important one, not the diastolic pressure. It's helpful to identify the brachial artery near the small groove at the medial edge of the distal biceps muscle; you should be able to palpate the artery here, and it's easier if the elbow is completely extended. Place the cuff high up on the upper limb **aligning the air bladder** (indicated on the cuff by an arrow) **over the brachial artery**. When you look at the cuff on the arm, approximately two- thirds of it should be encased, if not then a larger cuff may be required.

Now you're ready to **insonate the artery** with the handheld Doppler (insonate means to expose to ultrasound waves, that is, put the probe over the artery and turn it on). Now, about this machine – it's incredibly easy to use, don't be scared of it. It only has one button (on/off switch) and one dial (volume control) – that's it, you don't have to be a professor of vascular surgery to use one. **Turn the machine on** and cover the end of the transducer with **ultrasound gel**. Place the end over the artery facing into the anticipated direction of flow with a **45–60°** angle. You will know when you have found the artery because you will hear a distinctive pulsating sound, if you accidentally find a vein the sound could be described as similar to a windy storm. You may need to search a little to hear the sound clearly and in order to do so track the beam across the anticubital fossa medially or laterally (see the following Tip textbox for more on finding the arteries). Whilst you're principally concerned with the presence or absence of an arterial sound for the ABPI, it's also very helpful to understand the sound you're listening to, also called the waveform – see later for more details. Please also note that the final ABPI result will be based on the assumption that the brachial systolic pressure is representative of the systemic pressure, therefore if the brachial artery waveform is not normal (for example if the patient has a subcla-

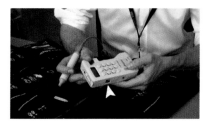

This is the handheld Doppler machine with an arrow pointing to the volume control. His thumb is on the on/off button

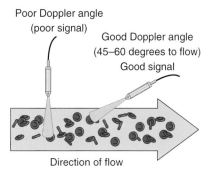

The optimal angle for Doppler insonation

vian artery stenosis) then it's a good idea to check the opposite brachial pressure and waveform and make a note of both readings, taking the highest as the most representative of the systemic pressure.

Now you're ready to **inflate the blood pressure cuff** and occlude the artery. Whilst pumping try to keep the probe completely still to avoid losing the signal. Just before the artery occludes there is often a 'whoosh' sound, which will give you a clue as to whether you've slipped off the artery. It's easy to slip off the artery – if you do don't worry just release some of

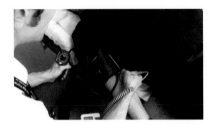

One hand pumps up the sphygmomanometer, the other holds the Doppler probe in position. Looking slick at doing all of this takes more practice than you think

Tip

Finding the arteries

1 **Do not move the probe too quickly** as you may skim over the artery in diastole and not hear the signal

2 Try to use your mind's eye to imagine the beam coming from the transducer. It will help you search for those elusive signals and help you to avoid making rapid sweeping movements by angling the probe too quickly

3 Making **very fine adjustments** in angle and probe location once a signal has been found will allow you to **optimise the sound** thus facilitate waveform identification and also help you to realise when you are slipping off the artery when inflating the cuff

the air from the cuff and readjust the probe until the signal returns, then adjust a little more so the signal is optimised. Once you can no longer hear a signal, the artery is occluded, **inflate for a further 20–30 mmHg** to ensure it is completely occluded. Now the cuff should be **deflated**, but slowly, around **2 mmHg per heartbeat** to ensure accuracy of the measurement. When the systolic blood pressure is reached the signal should return suddenly; at this point **make a note of the pressure**. The pressure usually returns a little lower than where it disappeared on inflation; it is this deflationary number you're interested in. Finally you should gradually release the cuff to restore blood flow to the arm. You're now ready to **take the ankle pressure.**

The ankle pressure is taken from two of the three main arteries supplying blood to the foot: the **dorsalis pedis artery (DPA)** and the **posterior tibial artery (PTA)** (the third is the peroneal artery but you don't use this for the ABPI). The DPA can be located running just laterally to the extensor hallucis longus tendon on the proximal half of the dorsal foot surface. The PTA is usually found just behind the medial malleolus. Now apply the cuff, it should be positioned so that the **bottom of the cuff is just above malleolar level**. Make sure that the **edges of the cuff are parallel rather than skewed**. What this means is that even if the leg is not cylindrical (which of course it rarely is), the cuff still should be, even if it means that it leaves a free space at the bottom of the cuff. Check the size is correct (i.e. two-thirds of the leg completely encased). When the cuff is applied properly take and record the pressures in the same way as for the brachial artery, remembering to use the same technique described above for finding the arteries.

Now you have all the systolic blood pressure readings it's time to **work out the**

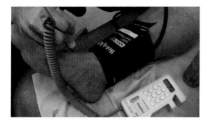

The dorsalis pedis artery

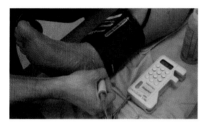

The posterior tibial artery

ABPI. The **highest pressure of the two arteries in each foot** is used in the calculation, you can discard the lower number:

$$ABPI = \frac{Ankle\,pressure\,(mm\,Hg)}{Brachial\,pressure\,(mm\,Hg)}$$

The following table gives an idea of the meaning of the ABPI clinically:

Resting ABPI	Disease severity
1.4 or greater	Calcification likely
0.9–1.3	Not suggestive of arterial disease
0.5–0.89	Suggests minor arterial disease (likely causing claudication)
0.49–0.3	Severe occlusive disease
Less than 0.3	Critical ischaemia with likely rest pain and tissue loss

Other notes

Waveforms

In some patients the lower limb arteries may become **calcified** due to disease, this is particularly common in patients with diabetes and chronic kidney failure. The calcification causes the arteries to stiffen and hence they will compress at a higher pressure than the true pressure **leading to an artifactually raised** ABPI. This is important to know as it means that in a diabetic patient with an ABPI of 0.8, it may in fact realistically be more like 0.4, the difference of which has clinical significance (see table). Luckily for us there is another way to assess whether there is healthy blood flow, by using the sound of the arterial pulse from the handheld Doppler otherwise known as the arterial waveforms.

There are three main types of arterial waveform, represented as different audible sounds:

- **Triphasic**: Each pulse has three phases to it, a large higher pitch sound followed by a lower pitch sound then a second higher pitch sound which is often quieter and lower than the original. This is the sound of a normal healthy artery.
- **Biphasic**: Each pulse has two phases a higher pitch followed by a lower pitch. Biphasic flow is often found in patients with minor peripheral arterial disease, or it can be normal.
- **Monophasic**: Each pulse has one phase to it, this is seen in severe cases

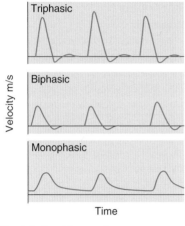

Triphasic

Biphasic

Monophasic

Velocity m/s

Time

Visual display of the waveforms

of peripheral arterial disease. The sound may be described as either **pulsatile** or **damped**.

- **Absent**: Due to occlusion of the artery, or occasionally congenital absence (approx 2–3% of the population for the DPA for example).

If a patient has a waveform which suggests peripheral arterial disease but a normal ABPI, the result should be considered suspiciously. However patients with an **ABPI ≥ 1.4 are considered to have diffusely calcified arteries** which may or may not be clinically symptomatic.

OSCE checklist

- Assembles equipment correctly
- Positions patient correctly
- Exposes limbs
- Applies BP cuff to arm
- Applies ultrasound gel to probe or artery
- Insonates brachial artery
- Inflates the BP cuff until the signal disappears
- Inflates by a further 20–30 mmHg
- Deflates gradually and notes systolic
- Applies BP cuff to ankle
- Applies gel over probe or artery
- Insonates dorsalis pedis
- Inflates BP cuff until signal disappears
- Inflates by a further 20–30 mmHg
- Deflates gradually and notes systolic
- Repeats with posterior tibial artery
- Repeats with the other leg
- Wipes off gel and advises to re-dress
- Calculates ABPI
- Washes hands
- Thanks patient
- Documents procedure
- Provides postprocedure advice

2   Arterial Blood Gas

Arthee Yogendran

Video Time | 2 mins 10 s

Overview

An arterial blood gas (or simply 'ABG') is exactly what it says on the tin: a blood sample taken from an artery. The benefits of an arterial sample as opposed to a venous sample is that you can find out the patient's level of blood oxygenation – arterial oxygen tension P_aO_2, as well as pH and arterial carbon dioxide levels P_aCO_2. Other benefits include a 'quick look' at electrolytes such as K+, haemoglobin levels and lactate, as opposed to waiting hours for the lab to process a venous blood sample. An arterial blood gas is perfect for rapidly identifying potentially reversible causes of acute problems allowing them to be addressed immediately, which may change the outcome of a desperate situation.

Commonly, the sample is taken from the radial artery. However, in situations such as the arrested/sick patient, the femoral artery is more likely to be successful – the hip is more stable, particularly during chest compressions and anatomically, the femoral artery is a bigger vessel than the radial artery. Therefore it's a larger target. Once the blood is obtained it needs to be heparinised to prevent it clotting en route to the analyser. Most hospitals now have specific ABG syringe packs, with prefilled heparin. Remember to discard the excess heparin to avoid a potentially diluted result. The heparin is merely there to line the collection apparatus to prevent the sample clotting and avert you pushing clots through an expensive analyser.

Before you take an ABG sample you should think about whether your patient may have any contraindications. Steer well clear if you can feel a thrill over that lump in the arm that actually, now you think about it looks a bit like a fistula. Avoid areas of infection, deformity or breaches to the skin. Also look out for any scars which depict

How to Perform Clinical Procedures, First Edition. Matthew Stephenson, Joshua Shur and John Black.
© 2013 John Wiley & Sons, Ltd. Published 2013 by John Wiley & Sons, Ltd.

previous surgery. The consultant vascular surgeon will not be overly impressed if you roger a recently placed bypass graft. Equally, watch out for groin hernias. A bowel puncture is generally best avoided. Finally, if you're contemplating a radial artery stab, it's important to assess your patient's collateral ulnar arterial supply using **Allen's test**, as should the radial artery thrombose following puncture, you may render them with an ischaemic hand if their collateral vasculature is poor.

Indications	Contraindications	Complications
Many! But broadly to: • Identify acid-base abnormalities • Identify severity of respiratory disease	• Ipsilateral arteriovenous fistula (for dialysis) • Local infection over puncture site • Large hernia (for femoral puncture) • Failure to fill hand by ulnar artery (Allen's test)	• Thrombosis • Dissection • Pseudoaneurysm • Haemorrhage • Peripheral ischaemia (rare)

Procedure

Make sure you have the **correct patient**, for the **correct procedure**. Check for any **allergies** (e.g. to the plaster you're going to put on at the end), and that you have confirmed the **indication;** excluded any **contraindications; explained** the procedure and taken **consent**. Now **wash your hands**!

Assemble all of your equipment on a trolley away from the patient. You will need everything in the equipment textbox. Remember to **discard the millilitre or so of the prefilled heparin** from the syringe to avoid a diluted sample result.

Have a feel of the **radial pulse** in one arm. If palpable, the radial artery is preferable to the femoral artery as it's more superficial. Palpate gently as you may

unintentionally occlude the artery, falsely convincing yourself of an absent pulse. The artery should be more superficial distally and thus an easier target. **Perform Allen's test** (see following textbox), which is a simple way of checking the adequacy of the collateral supply of blood to the hand.

Equipment you need (on a sterile tray/trolley)

- ABG pack containing:
  - Syringe prefilled with heparin
  - Needle (23G, Blue)
  - Cap (to cover the syringe after use)
- Alcohol wipe (or other sterile wipe)
- Sterile gauze
- Tape to secure gauze
- Gloves (non-sterile)
- A sharps bin

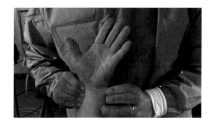

Allen's test being performed. The doctor's left hand has just released the pressure over the ulna artery and the palm's colour has restored

If a radial pulse is ambiguous or in an **emergency** situation, the **femoral artery offers an acceptable alternative**. Rather than just rummaging around trying to locate a femoral pulse somewhere in the region of the patient's genitals, let's look back at our anatomy. The femoral artery is found at the **mid-inguinal point** or midway between the symphysis pubis and anterior superior iliac spine. These are your bony landmarks. It's worth noting that the femoral vein lies just medial to your target – a useful mnemonic is NAVY (progressing lateral to medial): Femoral nerve, artery, vein, and finally 'Y' fronts depending on the gender of your patient. During an arrest it's best to try to obtain your sample during chest compressions if possible so you have the benefit of a pulse actually being palpable or at least a 1/3 of a stroke volume filling the vessel assuming that your colleague's chest compressions are effective.

For radial samples **position the forearm supinated** and **dorsiflex the wrist** to 40°. After **cleaning the area** of intended puncture with an alcohol-based wipe, with your gloved non-dominant hand, palpate the pulse and warn the patient of an impending sharp prick. Holding the syringe in your dominant hand **advance the needle** (bevel up) towards the pulse at a 30–45° angle to the skin, anchoring the overlying skin and subcutaneous tissues with your non-dominant hand just proximal to your needle insertion site.

Be patient, often you won't get the sample immediately. Arteries can be more tortuous and mobile in the elderly for instance. Once through the skin, stop and re-palpate the pulse. If you're still in the line of the artery, try going deeper, otherwise a small change of direction medially or laterally, can give you the flash-back you crave. Remember that you can often find the artery this way without the needle even completely exiting the skin. Make slow

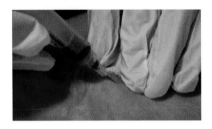

The needle is advanced at about 30° and blood rapidly starts to fill the syringe

advances so you don't end up going through the artery. If you had flash back and now your syringe has ceased filling, you have probably gone through the artery to the other side. Try withdrawing slightly. If you're in the artery, the **syringe should fill independently under arterial pressure** (although some ABG syringes are not designed like this, you have to aspirate yourself, check your own trust's syringes). Additionally, the blood is a rich oxygenated colour as opposed to darker venous blood. If you're using a non-filling syringe or if the patient is hypotensive, pull back gently on the plunger to aspirate your sample. Again, check whether your sample looks dark, as this could indicate a venous or mixed sample. You'll soon know if the oxygen saturations processed are only 67% (indicating venous blood or a very sick patient)!

Once you have collected about 3–5 mls of blood, **remove the needle** and apply the **gauze with firm pressure** over the puncture site. If it's a femoral stab, you should sit there for at least 10–15 minutes applying pressure – femoral pseudoaneurysms do happen, and the vascular surgeon will be less than happy to have to come and fix the hole in the artery. Drop the **needle straight into the sharps bin** and put the cap on the syringe. Make sure you **remove any air bubbles**, and **make a note of the amount of oxygen therapy** the patient has been receiving, and their temperature. Noting the temperature ensures the analyser calculates the correct partial pressure. **Transport your sample promptly** to an analyser for processing, these are usually found in the intensive care unit or emergency department.

Don't throw away the remnants of your sample in the syringe until you have fed the analyzer and have a legible **printed result** in your hand. Sometimes, a system or technical error occurs and you may need to run a repeat analysis for whatever frustrating reason. It would mean having to repeat the puncture. Fishing your sample from a bin full of sharps is dangerous – never do it. Remember to collect the paper print out of your analysis. Ensure that the result is **dated and timed**, with the correct patient details and that the amount of oxygen they were inspiring is clearly recorded and put this into the patient's notes. It's preferable to also write the results in the notes, as results that are stuck in have a tendency to become un-stuck!

OSCE checklist
- Assembles equipment correctly
- Disposes of excess heparin
- Correctly performs Allen's test
- Dons gloves
- Cleans area
- Positions wrist
- Palpates the radial pulse
- Warns about a 'sharp scratch'
- Inserts needle at approximately 20–30°
- If necessary repositions needle
- Watches for flashback
- Obtains sample successfully
- Withdraws needle and applies pressure
- Disposes of sharp immediately
- Places cap or bung on syringe
- Notes inspired oxygen concentration and body temperature
- Promptly analyses blood
- Washes hands
- Thanks patient
- Documents procedure
- Provides postprocedure advice

3 Arterial Cannulation

Reshma Woograsingh and Christopher Parnell

Video Time | 3 mins 4 s

Overview

Arterial cannulation is most commonly used in the intensive care/high dependency setting and is often used in theatre as well. It enables an invasive form of blood pressure monitoring that allows rapid assessment of blood pressure 'beat-to-beat', rather than waiting for an automated blood pressure cuff to inflate and deflate a few times only to show an error message – not so good in a sick patient! The advantages of this method of monitoring are pretty clear for patients who are on rapidly acting vasoactive medication and as an F1/2 working in intensive care/high dependency it's a pretty good skill to have. Another advantage is that arterial blood gas measurements can be taken from the arterial line thereby avoiding further punctures to your patient. It is, however, not without risk and in the following table are a few things to consider before going ahead with this procedure.

Procedure

Make sure you have the **correct patient**, for the **correct procedure**. Check for any **allergies**, and that you have confirmed the **indication;** excluded any **contraindications; explained** the procedure and taken **consent**. Now **wash your hands**!

The site of insertion of an arterial cannula is most often the radial artery. However, other sites include the femoral, brachial and dorsalis pedis. An **Allen's test** can help identify collateral flow from the ulnar artery to supply the palmar arch. Ask the patient to elevate their hand and **occlude both the radial and ulnar arteries**. Next, ask the patient to **form a fist** for a few seconds before opening their palm – their hand should appear blanched. Finally, **release the pressure on the ulnar**

How to Perform Clinical Procedures, First Edition. Matthew Stephenson, Joshua Shur and John Black.
© 2013 John Wiley & Sons, Ltd. Published 2013 by John Wiley & Sons, Ltd.

Indications	Contraindications	Complications
• Monitoring arterial blood pressure whilst on inotropes/vasopressors • Monitoring arterial blood gas measurements in high dependency / critical care – this also allows for frequent blood sampling without venepuncture • General anaesthesia cases where there may be rapid swings in blood pressure • When non-invasive blood pressure is inadequate/fails, e.g obese patients undergoing prolonged general anaesthesia	• Absence of pulse • Localised infection over intended insertion site • Prior surgery in the region, eg. Vascular graft • Bleeding diathesis (relative) • Negative Allen's test implying no collateral flow from ulnar artery to palmar arch (relative)	• Arterial thrombosis/ ischaemia • Haematoma at insertion site • Arteriovenous fistula formation • Pseudoaneurysm formation • Infection/sepsis • Nerve injury

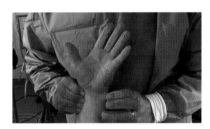

Allen's test being performed. The ulnar artery has just been released and the palm is pinking up

Equipment you need (on a sterile tray/trolley)

- Arterial cannula, e.g. 20G Floswitch
- Skin preparation, e.g. Chlorhexidine
- Local anaesthetic, e.g. lidocaine
- Sterile gauze
- 2 ml syringe for local anaesthetic
- 10 ml syringe with normal saline connected to three-way tap and short extension (usually the distal end of transducer set)
- Sterile dressing +/– bio-occlusive dressing

artery, there should be rapid flow and hyperaemia of the palm, indicating good flow from that ulnar artery.

Assemble all of your equipment on a sterile trolley away from the patient. You will need everything in the equipment textbox.

The technique of placing a Floswitch type of arterial cannula is known as a 'catheter-over-needle' method, which is very similar to cannulating a peripheral vein. The procedure should be performed in an aseptic manner and some units advocate not only using sterile gloves and drapes, but even require full surgical attire to perform this task.

Position is key to your success – have the **arm abducted** onto a pillow at their side and ask the patient to have their **wrist slightly cocked back**. This helps to stabilise the radial artery. If you are fortunate to have an assistant, they can help to hold the fingertips and stabilise the forearm. Alternatively, you may find that placing their wrist on top of a bag of intravenous fluid (wrapped in a pillowcase) and some strategically placed tape on the fingers to the bed is all that is required.

Prepare the area with a suitable cleaning solution- this time we have used chlorhexidine. A sterile drape may come in handy here to ensure a sterile field. For the purposes of demonstration we have left the area visible. **Local anaesthetic** can be infiltrated at the intended insertion site. Only a small amount is needed, say 1 ml of 1% lidocaine. It's not always used however, even in awake patients.

With one hand, **palpate the artery** just proximal to the flexor palmar crease and imagine the course of the artery as you feel it. Holding the cannula in the other hand attempt to puncture the artery; the angle between the cannula and the skin should be **20–30°**. Hopefully you will see flashback of blood into the cannula indicating that the needle is in the artery. If not, withdraw the needle and cannula slightly within the skin and redirect.

One tip here is that once you have obtained good flashback, **advance the cannula a further 1–2 mm** to ensure its tip is within the artery – at this point only the bevel of the needle is definitely in the vessel.

Hold the needle steady and slide the cannula into the artery – don't force it! Or else you will create a false passage. Never reinsert the needle into the cannula – this could cause shearing of the line. **Remove the needle** and attach the line to the primed end of a transducer set. This is often a syringe of saline attached to a 3-way tap on a short 100 mm extension. The trans-

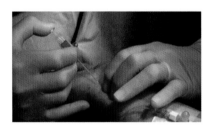

The fingers of the non-dominant hand are palpating the line of the artery and the needle is angled for approach

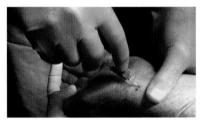

The cannula has been inserted, the needle is being withdrawn and the switch is about to be turned off

ducer set is different to other giving sets in that the tubing is more rigid than a standard 3-way tap on an extension. This minimises disruption of the transducer reading from the arterial pulsation. The sets are also often distinguished by a longitudinal red stripe so as to highlight the fact that it is connected to an artery.

Confirm **easy aspiration of arterial blood** and smooth, **easy flushing of saline** before removing the drapes, cleaning the area and **securing with a sterile dressing**. There are also purpose-made anchoring dressings available for this too. A clear, occlusive dressing should be applied over the insertion site as well.

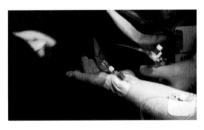

The dressings applied to secure the arterial cannula

There are often special arterial line alert stickers that can be placed on the dressing. **Dispose of your sharps** (including the guidewire) immediately into a sharps bin. **Document the procedure** clearly in the notes.

A quick word about types of arterial cannulae

You will notice that the one in the video is called a Floswitch, which has the advantage of being able to be locked off quickly after insertion. There are other brands and types available. One other popular technique uses a 20G Vygon Leader-Cath.

This adopts the Seldinger technique, which is a 'catheter-over-wire' technique that is the same method as is often used when putting in a central line. A needle introducer is inserted to find the artery, sometimes with a 2 ml syringe attached to store any flashback. Once located, the syringe is removed and a guidewire is passed through the needle. The needle is then removed to leave only the wire lying in the artery. The next step is to introduce the catheter over the wire, keeping a hold of the distal end so as not to lose the guidewire (unlike the central line, there is no need to dilate). Finally the wire is removed leaving the cannula in place ready to be attached to the saline syringe with extension. As before, checks for easy aspiration of arterial blood and flushing are performed.

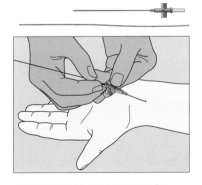

An illustration of the catheter-over-wire technique

OSCE checklist

- Assembles equipment correctly
- Correctly performs Allen's test
- Scrubs and dons appropriate sterile personal protective attire
- Cleans skin
- Positions wrist
- Palpates the radial pulse
- Warns about a 'sharp scratch'
- Injects local anaesthetic superficial to artery
- Angulates needle at approximately 20–30°
- Watches for flashback
- If necessary repositions needle (without exiting skin)
- Advances the cannula
- Compresses the artery proximally
- Withdraws the needle
- Closes the cannula with the locking device
- Attaches the cannula to a saline flush
- Re-opens the arterial cannula
- Aspirates to check placement, then flushes
- Closes the arterial cannula switch again
- Secures the cannula with dressings
- Washes hands
- Thanks patient
- Disposes of sharps and waste
- Documents procedure
- Provides postprocedure advice

4 Ascitic Drain

Video Time | 4 mins 15 s

Overview

Ascitic drainage is a therapeutic procedure designed to remove abdominal **ascites**. Unlike an ascitic tap, this procedure is used for **treatment rather than diagnosis**. It's a relatively quick and simple procedure and those who have spent some time on a gastroenterology firm will know that patients obtain quick relief from the procedure. Witnessing the sight of your patient staggering in sheer discomfort as they carry their hugely distended abdomens indicates how distressing massive ascites can be. Some patients arrive at hospital in desperation to have their ascites removed.

For junior doctors, therapeutic paracentesis is likely to become more common with the increasing prevalence of all forms of chronic liver disease (alcoholic liver disease, viral liver disease and fatty liver disease) and **ascites is the most common presentation of cirrhosis**. It's fair to say that most junior doctors who cover an acute medical take will have the opportunity to place at least one. It's technically not a demanding procedure however entering the abdomen is not without risks and so care needs to be taken when performing it. There are lots of important organs in there and the aim is to avoid them at all costs!

Although not exclusively due to cirrhosis, about 75% of cases of ascites are due to this. The cause for the development of ascites is complex but occurs as a result of liver fibrosis and the effect of vasoactive mediators resulting in a positive sodium balance. The development of ascites itself is a worrying sign and overall statistically a patient with ascites will have a 50% chance of dying at 2 years.

The British Society of Gastroenterology (BSG) guidelines advocate a stepwise approach to the treatment of ascites. Management starts with **salt restriction**

How to Perform Clinical Procedures, First Edition. Matthew Stephenson, Joshua Shur and John Black.
© 2013 John Wiley & Sons, Ltd. Published 2013 by John Wiley & Sons, Ltd.

(no added salt diet) and **diuretics** for small to moderate ascites. Patients who do not respond to these treatments and develop gross ascites are termed refractory and undergo repeat planned paracentesis. Those patients whose index presentation is with gross ascites would proceed directly to paracentesis and then their response to salt restriction and diuretics assessed. The decision is simpler if you have a patient presenting with massive ascites – there is no point in waiting weeks for a diuretic to work and you are much better off going straight for a drain. If the patient is intolerant of diuretics (hyponatraemia or rising creatinine), then repeat paracentesis would also be an option.

Indications	Contraindications	Complications
• The removal of large volumes of ascites refractory to diuretics (> 4 litres)	• Pregnancy • Bowel distension • Renal failure* • Coagulopathy* • Subacute bacterial peritonitis* • Hypotension* • Thrombocytopenia • Hepatic encephalopathy* (all relative)	• Bleeding/ Haemoperitoneum** • Visceral damage*** • Infection**** • Ascitic leak*****

*There have been no studies to support these, that said most physicians would weigh up the risks and benefits in performing paracentesis in these patients.
**Many cirrhotic patients have a baseline coagulopathy and thrombocytopenia BUT the incidence of significant bleeding is low provided the creatinine is not grossly elevated. Check their clotting before starting the procedure – that includes their platelet count.
***Visceral damage and perforation are rare, particularly if anatomical landmarks are carefully followed and/or ultrasound is used.
****Ascitic leak can be controlled by placing a suture, although most people don't do this. Placing a stoma bag over the site is often sufficient.
*****Infection is minimised by keeping the drain in for a short duration, less than 6 hours; leaving a drain in overnight is not recommended.

Procedure

Ascitic drains are normally placed in **either lower abdominal quadrant** to ensure you avoid the large, more fixed solid organs, that is, liver and spleen. Remember that many patients with ascites will have hepatomegaly or hepato-splenomegaly and as such it's extremely **important to examine** your patient before starting the procedure, to identify the lower edges of these organs. A quick look at any recent ultrasound or CT scans is more often useful because with gross ascites palpating any organs can be difficult.

In tense ascites it will be fairly clear where the fluid is located. For patients with more moderate ascites then it can be difficult. With the patient supine, rolling them to one side helps the fluid to collect. Ultrasound can also locate the ascites-but usually it is clinically apparent where the fluid is if a patient requires a drain. In complicated patients, for instance where there are scars indicating previous surgery (and hence the possibility of adhesions of bowel to the abdominal wall), ultrasound guided drainage should be used.

Make sure you have the **correct patient**, for the **correct procedure**. Check for any **allergies**, and that you have confirmed the **indication;** excluded any **contraindications; explained** the procedure and taken **consent**. Now **wash your hands**!

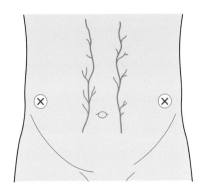

The X marks the point of maximal safety for needle entry

Assemble all of your equipment on a sterile trolley away from the patient.

Equipment you need (on a sterile tray/trolley)

- Sterile dressing pack including:
  - Sterile drape
  - Sterile gauze
  - Sterile gloves
- Blue needle (23G)
- Green needle (21G)
- 20 ml syringes
- 10 ml syringe
- Local anaesthetic (e.g. 10 ml lidocaine)
- Bonanno catheter including catheter bag attachment
- Catheter drainage bag
- Adhesive dressing
- Specimen pots
- Cleaning solution

You will need everything in the equipment textbox. This procedure is strictly **aseptic** and so it's important to maintain a sterile field.

Position your patient in the **supine** position and make sure they're **comfortable, with an empty bladder**, and rest their head on a pillow. It's useful to **mark** where you will insert the drain before starting. A typical point would be placed **on a line from umbilicus to the**

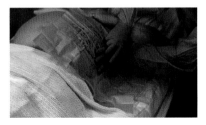

Confirmation of site of planned drainage by testing dullness to percussion

anterior superior iliac spine (ASIS) where percussion is dullest. Some people find it easier to mark the planned point of drain insertion.

At this point you should put on your **sterile gloves and apron**. The Bonanno catheter should be assembled prior to starting. It will come as the curled drain, guide needle and sheath. Firstly **uncurl the catheter** by moving the sheath along it. When it's straight **insert the needle** as far as possible. The **outer sheath can then be removed** so that the drain is held straight over the guide needle. Don't insert the needle until the drain is straight or the needle

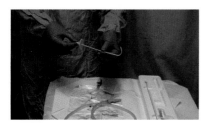

This is the Bonanno catheter, the left hand is sliding the sheath along the catheter to straighten it out

will cut through the drain. It's worth pointing out that Bonanno catheters are not the only drain used for ascites and were not actually originally manufactured for ascitic drainage.

Once the insertion site is marked it can be **cleaned** using your hospital's usual skin cleaning solution and then **sterile drapes** are placed. Infiltrate the subcuta-

neous tissue with **local anaesthetic**, and then perpendicular to the epidermis into the deeper tissues in the line of the intended passage of the ascitic drain. In total approximately 5–10 mls of lidocaine should suffice. Make a **very small incision** with a scalpel over your bleb because this allows the drain to penetrate the tough skin without excessive pressure.

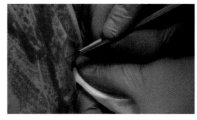

Once local anaesthetic is in, make a small stab incision for the skin only

Now you're ready to **insert the needle** (with Bonanno drain held straight over it). Hold the drain in your dominant hand and **advance a few millimetres at a time aspirating as you go**. Many clinicians recommend a 'Z' track which involves puncturing the skin perpendicularly, the subcutaneous tissues and muscles obliquely and then perpendicularly through the peritoneum. When the drain is removed the remaining tissue tract should then close spontaneously reducing the chance of a leak.

When the needle reaches the peritoneal cavity you may feel a sudden loss of resistance and on suction ascitic

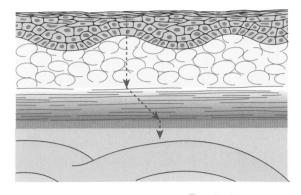

	Skin
	Subcutaneous tissue + muscle
	Peritoneum
	Ascites

The z-tract

fluid will enter the syringe. This is when you should **collect your samples** if indicated. **Advance the needle** approximately 1 more centimetre to ensure that the drain is in the correct space. Whilst **keeping the drain still withdraw the needle and simultaneously advance the cannula** until the flange of the drain meets the skin. As you do so the cannula will curl into place in the peritoneal cavity. **Attach the catheter bag** attachment and then the catheter bag and it should start to drain freely.

Note, the ascites can be under quite high pressure so **make sure the clamp is closed** on the bag attachment. An apron or gown can save a trip to the dry cleaners but there are no words to describe walking around in socks that are saturated with someone else's bodily fluids: Be ready to put your finger over the end of the catheter. Occasionally fluid may not drain, this can be due to poor choice of site, loculated ascites, overlying omentum or a small clot in the

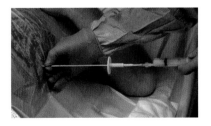

The needle has entered the peritoneal cavity and fluid is being aspirated from the syringe, confirming position

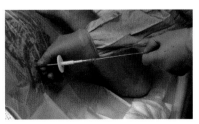

The catheter is advanced over the needle

cannula. As a last resort it may be necessary to re-site the drain to the other side of the abdomen.

The **drain can then be secured** in place with sterile gauze to pad around the catheter covered in sterile transparent dressings, suturing is not recommended.

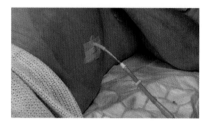

The drain is secured with simple adhesive dressings

It's usually advised to remove the drain after about 6 hours. This will minimise the chance of secondary bacterial infection. **To remove the drain**, the dressings are peeled off and then the catheter is gently pulled out. The drain site can be covered with some gauze and another adhesive dressing.

As with any procedure it's important to **fully document** what you've done and in addition to the usual things you'd write, comment on whether the ascites was bloody and also when the drain should be removed.

Finally make sure you have prescribed the **volume replacement regime** (see the following textbox) and handed over for the drain to be removed if this won't be you. If you are sending samples to the lab then you should make sure you have filled out the request form correctly. Samples should be sent for cell count, M, C & S, amylase, albumin and protein. If you are suspecting a malignant ascites then you can send your sample for further tests including cytology.

To volume replace or not volume replace?

Current guidelines recommend the use of volume replacement after completing drainage of large amounts of fluid, simply because it's safer and more effective. There is a risk that by removing large amounts of fluid from the intra-abdominal space without any volume replacement, the resulting circulatory changes can cause renal dysfunction, electrolyte disturbance and hypotension. Current best practice recommends:

- For paracentesis of <5 L volume replace with a synthetic plasma expander such as gelofusin, depending on patient observations.
- For paracentesis of >5 L volume replace with albumin. A rough guide would be approximately 100mls of 20% human albumin solution for every 2.5 L drained.

OSCE checklist

- Examines the patient to identify site of drainage
- Assembles equipment correctly
- Scrubs and dons appropriate sterile personal protective attire
- Selects site for puncture
- Cleans skin
- Applies aperture drape
- Confirms dullness to percussion
- Checks local anaesthetic
- Warns about a 'sharp scratch'
- Injects local anaesthetic superficial (e.g. lidocaine 2%)
- Performs diagnostic tap (optional)
- Straightens catheter with sleeve
- Inserts needle
- Removes sleeve
- Attaches 5 ml syringe
- Closes drain connector
- Makes a nick in the skin with the blade
- Handles the needle and catheter safely
- Advances needle slowly whilst aspirating
- Withdraws fluid to confirm correct position
- Advances catheter, keeping needle still
- Removes needle
- Attaches connector (closed)
- Attaches drainage bag
- Opens connector
- Secures with dressings or suture
- Washes hands
- Thanks patient
- Disposes of sharps and waste
- Documents procedure
- Provides postprocedure advice

5 Ascitic Tap

Video Time | 3 mins 58 s

Overview

Drawing off ascitic fluid for **diagnostic** purposes is a quick, easy and (usually) straightforward procedure. It can look a bit daunting at first, shoving a needle into someone's abdomen but with a bit of confidence it's an easy skill that any doctor or medical student can get the hang of.

'I thought we had already been through this,' I hear those who have just read the **Ascitic Drain** chapter say … close. What we are dealing with here is taking off only about 20–60 mls of fluid to **aid getting a diagnosis**. What kind of patients are we dealing with? Well, essentially *anyone* with **ascites**, especially when the underlying diagnosis is **unknown**.

With this in mind your typical patient will be encountered on the gastro, oncology or gynaecology wards and on the acute medical unit (AMU). It's also part of the 'package' when you might suspect someone has spontaneous bacterial peritonitis (SBP). So if you work in any of the above wards be ready to practise your technique!

Before explaining the procedure in more detail probably the main thing to emphasise is **placement** of your needle. This is key to reducing any possible complications and also to maximise your chance of getting fluid.

Some clinicians get very anxious when performing this procedure on patients with deranged clotting. These are generally **not** gastroenterologists. They will tell you that it's probably safe to proceed in most cases. This is simply because little evidence supports the contrary. Most gastroenterologists, however, would advocate a bit of haematological cover (for example vitamin K, FFP and if necessary platelets) for this procedure

How to Perform Clinical Procedures, First Edition. Matthew Stephenson, Joshua Shur and John Black.
© 2013 John Wiley & Sons, Ltd. Published 2013 by John Wiley & Sons, Ltd.

if the INR goes above 2 or the platelets drop below around 40 x 10^9/L, however correction is less important than when placing a drain. In fact complications with this procedure are rare – and with a green needle you are unlikely to do much damage.

Indications	Contraindications	Complications
• Ascites of unknown origin • Spontaneous bacterial peritonitis	Relative: • Bowel obstruction • Localised infection at puncture site • Severe bleeding diathesis – including coagulopathy and thrombocytopenia.	• Haematoma • Visceral damage (e.g. bowel perforation is very rare) • Bleeding/ haemoperitoneum

Procedure

Make sure you have the **correct patient**, for the **correct procedure**. Check for any **allergies**, and that you have confirmed the **indication;** excluded any **contraindications; explained** the procedure and taken **consent**. Now **wash your hands**!

Position your patient in the **supine** position and make sure they are **comfortable, have an empty bladder**, and rest their head on a pillow. **Assemble all of your equipment** on a trolley away from the patient. You will need everything in the equipment textbox. This procedure is strictly **aseptic** and so it's important to maintain a sterile field.

As for placing an ascitic drain the most important thing to do preprocedure is **examine** your patient. Look for any signs of organomegaly and percuss carefully for ascites. A recent CT or

> **Equipment you need (on a sterile tray/trolley)**
>
> • Green needle (21G)
> • 20 ml or 50 ml Luer lock syringe
> • Sterile pack containing:
>   ◦ Sterile gauze
>   ◦ Sterile gloves
>   ◦ Sterile drape
> • Local anaesthetic (optional)
> • Specimen bottles
> • Sterile cleaning swab
> • Adhesive dressing
> • Ultrasound probe (optional)
> • Sterile probe covers (optional)
> • Coupling media (ultrasound gel) (optional)

ultrasound can be a big help here. Some people like to **mark** the point where you are going to take the tap with a pen for example or make an indent in the skin.

The following figure shows the area where you want to aim for-avoiding the inferior epigastric arteries that run lateral to the umbilicus. Percuss from umbilicus to anterior superior iliac spine and where it is dullest should be the area you want to go for.

Once you have marked your area liberally **clean the skin** and then **drape** the abdomen. This can be a full drape or just a sterile sheet tucked underneath.

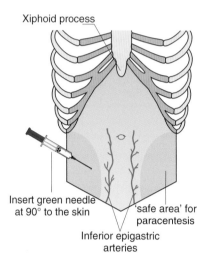

Xiphoid process

Insert green needle at 90° to the skin

'safe area' for paracentesis

Inferior epigastric arteries

The safe areas for paracentesis, avoiding the solid organs and abdominal wall vessels

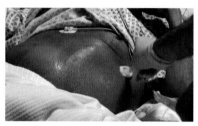

The abdomen is exposed and the skin is being cleaned here with an alcohol based skin prep

Ultrasound guidance

Bedside ultrasound enables you to tap much 'smaller' ascites (referring to your BSG guidelines you would know that this correlates with 'grade 1' ascites). In the DVD we show you how to do it with ultrasound and by all means go for it if you are used to this. With tense ascites, however, ultrasound isn't normally necessary.

Should you use local anaesthetic?

Many clinicians advocate doing this procedure without local. This is simply because local anaesthetic is painful, and if you do infiltrate first you will be using 2 needles instead of 1. In addition with ascites, the abdomen can be tense resulting in a 'squashed' abdominal wall to infiltrate. However other clinicians will say it's better to use local. This is because putting a needle into the body doesn't just hurt whilst it's inside you, it stings for a while afterwards, and whilst the injection of local is painful for a few seconds, it stops this prolonged post-needling sting. In the end it's up to you and your patient.

If you are using ultrasound, ensure that the probe has some jelly applied and a sterile cover wrapped around it.

Warn your patient of a **sharp sting** and slowly **insert the needle** perpendicular to the abdomen. Apply **gentle negative pressure** as you do so. In tense ascites you should start receiving fluid after only a few millimetres. If you don't get anything at first then don't panic, withdraw slightly and reposition the needle.

If you are the ultrasounding-type then you will be able to follow the needle as an

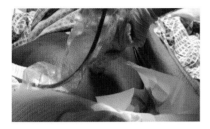

The ultrasound probe is positioned over the intended site of puncture, note the plastic sheath that covers it and its cable. Not everyone uses ultrasound

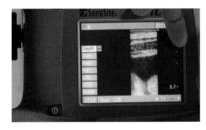

An image of the ultrasound picture. At the top is skin and below this are the layers of the abdominal wall. At the bottom, the two rounded shapes are bowel, and the large black area is your easy target: the ascites

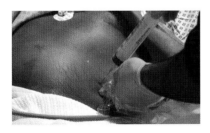

The needle is inserted at 90° to the skin and next to the probe, the tip can then be visualised on the screen

SAAG

The serum ascites-albumin gradient is a more accurate method of distinguishing the cause of ascites than the previously used **transudative** and **exudative**. Essentially you subtract the ascitic fluid albumin concentration from the serum albumin concentration. A gradient of >11 g/L (transudative) indicates that the cause is due to a portal hypertensive process including heart failure, Budd Chiari and cirrhosis. A gradient of <11 g/L (exudative) indicates portal hypertension is not a prominent cause and includes causes such as malignant ascites, peritoneal tuberculosis and pancreatitis. So when sending off your samples, make sure you remember to request an ascites albumin!

Aside from the SAAG, knowing the amylase can in selected cases be helpful: ascites can accumulate due to pancreatic inflammation so a huge amylase should alert you to this possibility.

acoustic tip as it enters the abdomen. Ensure you keep it next to the probe head as you image and again apply negative pressure to elicit fluid.

Once you have obtained enough fluid **remove the needle** and **apply pressure with some gauze** and then you can stick this down with an adhesive

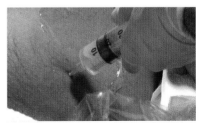

Straw coloured ascitic fluid withdrawn into the syringe

dressing. The sample can give you useful information just by looking at it macroscopically – is it purulent looking or clear/straw coloured? Is there blood? All of this can give you clues to its origin.

Once you have obtained your sample decant it into your specimen bottles as required. Basic investigations you should send for include:

- fluid protein/albumin (include a serum albumin if you need to calculate the SAAG – see the following textbox)
- amylase
- M, C and S
- cell count
- cytology (if suspicion of malignancy)

Once your samples are sent off you're nearly finished. Thank your patient and **document** the procedure in the notes-

particularly which investigations have been requested.

Spontaneous Bacterial Peritonitis (SBP)

This unfortunate complication of ascites is precisely as it sounds. Symptoms are often vague and might be interpreted as a gradual non-specific decline. Fever, pain, nausea, and vomiting are rare but deteriorating LFTs are common. Approximately 10% of 'ascitic' inpatients will suffer SBP.

SBP is the diagnosis if the ascitic neutrophil count level is above 250 cells/mm^3. If this result is not back before you go home, ask the on-call to check it and start them on antibiotics as required. A broad spectrum agent such as co-amoxiclav, ciprofloxacin or in some cases tazocin is usually preferred.

OSCE checklist

- Assembles equipment correctly
- Places patient in a supine position
- Examines the patient to confirm site of drainage
- Cleans area
- Places drapes
- Uses ultrasound correctly (if appropriate)
- Warns about a 'sharp scratch'
- Infiltrates local anaesthetic correctly
- Attaches syringe to needle
- Inserts needle perpendicular to skin
- Advances needle slowly whilst aspirating
- Aspirates sample successfully
- Removes needle and applies pressure with gauze
- Labels samples and completes request form correctly
- Washes hands
- Thanks patient
- Disposes of sharps and waste
- Documents procedure
- Provides postprocedure advice

6 Back Slab – Below Knee

Video Time | 3 mins 26 s

Overview

Whilst fractures are of course most commonly seen in A&E, they aren't usually definitively managed there. Some fractures require immediate admission and repair but the majority need some form of **temporary limb immobilisation** and an appointment for the fracture clinic. The task of this chapter is simply to show you how to provide said immobilisation, not to diagnose different types of fractures or other management algorithms.

As an orthopaedic surgical trainee or A&E frontman, you will unquestionably be called to plaster limbs, ankle injuries for instance account for about 5% of presentations to A&E. A&E nurses are almost invariably trained in plastering, thank goodness, but sometimes they'll be busier than you and it's quicker to simply do it yourself. Plus, what kind of an A&E/orthopaedic doctor are you if you can't even plaster a limb? It's one of those rites of passage as a doctor.

In A&E, plastering is best done with a **Plaster of Paris (POP) back slab**. It's simple to do and if the limb swells soon after the injury, it's not confined to a rigid circumferential case. More definitive casts can be made later after fracture clinic review and the swelling has gone down. The principles are similar for whichever limb fracture you're dealing with, but in this case we're focusing on the **ankle fracture**.

Procedure

Make sure you have the **correct patient**, for the **correct procedure**. Check for any **allergies**, and that you have confirmed the **indication;** excluded any **contraindications; explained** the procedure and taken **consent**. Now **wash your hands**!

How to Perform Clinical Procedures, First Edition. Matthew Stephenson, Joshua Shur and John Black.
© 2013 John Wiley & Sons, Ltd. Published 2013 by John Wiley & Sons, Ltd.

Indications	Contraindications	Complications
• Limb fractures that can wait until fracture clinic	• Fractures requiring urgent surgery such as open or unstable fractures • Intolerance to plaster of Paris (there are alternatives)	• Discomfort • Irritation to the skin • Cast tightening secondary to swelling • Cast loosening • DVT • Neurovascular compromise

Assemble all of your equipment on a trolley away from the patient. You will need everything in the equipment textbox and it all usually comes together on a dedicated plastering trolley. Warn the patient particularly that the lower limb back slab cast is **non-weight bearing**, further decisions regarding its management, including weight bearing status will be made at the fracture clinic.

Equipment you need (on a sterile tray/trolley)

- Bowl of warm water (for plaster soaking and washing off residue)
- Towel
- Tape measure (optional)
- Patient couch with leg extension +/– leg rest
- Plaster of Paris bandages (10–20 cm wide)
- Bandage scissors
- Crepe bandages (15 cm wide)
- Stockinette (7.5 cm wide)
- Underplast padding (15 cm wide)
- Adhesive tape (optional)
- Plastic apron and protective plastic sheeting
- Gloves
- Crutches

A back slab consists of **two main elements**: Firstly, a **stirrup** which is intended to immobilise the lateral movements of the ankle at both malleoli. Secondly, a broader, thicker **posterior aspect** is then added which prevents dorsiflexion and plantarflexion of the foot. Together they deliver **immobility in all directions** which is your ultimate aim.

As a general rule, a slab that is between **15 and 20 cm wide** is used for the **posterior** component (depending on the size of the patient) and the **stirrup** is fashioned from a **10 cm wide strip**. The patient should be positioned on an extendable couch, preferably with a leg rest. Note that **plaster is an irritant** when in direct contact with the skin. Adorn the patient with protective sheets over the areas you wish to keep clean or give them a plastic apron to wear.

Ideally, this is a **two-person procedure**, as positioning and maintenance of the position throughout is key. Unless otherwise instructed, the **ankle is positioned at 90°** with the **foot in a neutral**

position. An exception is if the patient has sustained an Achilles tendon injury, in which case the ankle is placed in equinus (plantar flexion).

In order to **ascertain the length** of the posterior slab **measure** from below the back of the knee (leaving enough room for articulation at the knee joint) down the back of the leg and under the foot to the tips of the toes. For the stirrup, measure from the sides, just below the knee down under the ankle to the opposing side.

Prepare the posterior slab by cutting **6–8 layers** of POP between 15 and 20 cm width. Both the width and the layers of plaster used depend upon the type of patient. Use a little common sense: For Mrs Frail-old-lady, who is relatively immobile, 6 layers shall suffice with a 15 cm width. Conversely, a buff athlete would require 8 layers of 20 cm width and so on and so forth… For the **stirrup, 4–6 layers** are cut to length in preparation.

Put on your **gloves** and don your very own **apron** – things are about to get messy! Ask your assistant to **hold the toes** of the foot with one hand and **support the back of the knee** with the other, with the **knee** held in approximately **15° of flexion**. This will allow the calf muscles to relax and the foot to assume the natural position.

The first layer is the **stockinette** – an elasticated little number that will stop the underplast padding irritating the skin and your patient reaching for a knitting needle. Starting at the toes, **roll this up the leg** towards the knee.

Cut the stockinette longer than the length you intend to plaster, as this will then fold back to protect the skin from the edges of the overlying padding and plaster.

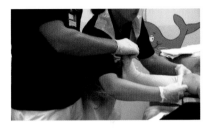

The stockinette is the first layer

Now you're ready for the under **cast-padding**. This is a synthetic material which cleverly accommodates swelling and reduces friction between the cast and the skin. Ideally it should be applied of a tension enough to take up any slack, but not too tight to obstruct venous return. There are no prizes for applying a tourniquet. Starting at the knee and working your way down, **apply** one layer towards the toes, doubling back on yourself with a second

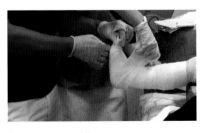

The undercast padding

layer over the bony prominences: The head of the fibula, the malleoli and the heel. As with the stockinette, remember to leave it longer than your intended plaster cast. Make sure positioning is maintained to avoid ruffling of the under-cast padding, which can lead to discomfort and your cast slipping.

Take one end of the **stirrup** length in each hand and **submerge it in the warm water** for approximately 4 seconds. Remove it from the bucket and squeeze out the excess fluid. **Fit the stirrup in a 'U' shape** flush with the heel up over each malleoli and each side of the leg. **Mould** the cast to the sides, smoothing out the plaster. **Shape it** over the malleoli (as these are the most mobile areas and require maximum support). Take extra care to make sure the plaster **does not meet anteriorly**.

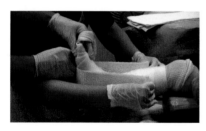

The U-shaped stirrup being measured before it is submerged in water

Next, take your 6–8 layers of carefully measured **posterior cast** and **submerge** it. As previously, squeeze out the excess water. Starting at the knee, place your plaster posteriorly towards the ankle and around the heel heading for the toes.

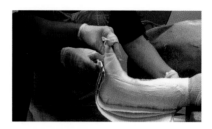

The posterior stirrup being measured before it's submerged in water

Mould the posterior slab around the shape of the calf and up around the malleoli to meet your stirrup slab. Using a similar action, bring the plaster up around the edges of the hallux and little toes. With **long sweeping actions**, **smooth the plaster** once positioned so it becomes as one entity. The cast should be firm to touch within the hour and dries completely at around 6 hours post application. **Wash off any plaster** which is on the patient's toes and probably your own arms and face depending on how much fun you had!

You're almost there. **Reflect the stockinette** and under-cast padding back on itself over your plaster cast (the excess which has been purposefully left) at both the knee and the toes. Finish by **applying the crepe bandage**, again starting at the knee and working distally towards the toes, trapping the reflected underlying layers neatly under the bandage. **Fix the end of the bandage** with strips of adhesive tape or small offcuts of wet plaster… and **_Voila!_** The job is done.

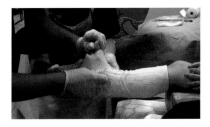

The stockinette is reflected back over the plaster

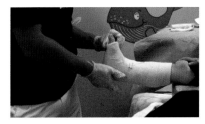

The finished product, with the crepe bandage wrapped around and a small offcut of wet plaster used to secure it

After **clearing up** all of your waste appropriately, check that the patient remains **neurovascularly intact** and test their **capillary refill time**. **Document** this carefully in the notes. **Counsel the patient** with regards to cast care and inform them of the clinical signs which may signify the cast is too tight. Make sure they have been **referred for follow up in fracture clinic**. This is usually in a few days, the A&E department usually has a protocol for deciding when certain fractures are due to come back. Supply the patient with a pair of **crutches to mobilise** and make sure they've been **properly taught how to use them**.

OSCE checklist

- Positions limb at appropriate angle
- Applies stockinette
- Applies undercast padding
- Maintains position
- Prepares plaster for stirrup
- Moulds stirrup to lateral and medial borders
- Ensures correct consistency
- Measures and prepares back slab
- Moulds back slab posteriorly
- Trims and reflects stockinette
- Applies crêpe bandage
- Secures with adhesive strip/tape
- Documents neurovascular status
- Washes hands
- Thanks patient
- Documents procedure
- Provides postprocedure advice

7 Back Slab – Upper Limb

Sarah Fisher

Video Time | 6 mins 6 s

Overview

As an A+E staff member, one of the most frequent bony injuries you will be asked to see is a fractured distal radius, such as a Colles' fracture requiring application of a back slab plaster cast. The commonest mechanism of injury is a FOOSH or 'Fall On Out Stretched Hand'. The back slab ensures that the wrist is immobilised yet allows enough room to accommodate any subsequent swelling of the forearm.

Whilst most departments have trained nurses for plaster application, it's always useful to know how to apply a temporary cast yourself. This video focuses on fashioning a back slab, so that you can safely send your patient home confident in the knowledge that you've adequately immobilised their injury until they are seen in fracture clinic, where the orthopaedic surgeons will be left blinded by your plastering skills (it really doesn't take that much to impress an orthopod).

Indications	Contraindications	Complications

• Fracture/dislocation:
  ∘ Distal radius/ulnar
  ∘ Carpal bones
  ∘ Metacarpals
   (if displaced)
	• Gross swelling
	• Skin breach/open
	  fracture
	• Injury requiring ORIF
	  (Open Reduction
	  Internal Fixation)
		• Skin irritation/dermatitis
		• Reduced dexterity (temporary)
		• Cast tightening
		• Joint stiffness (following
		  removal)

How to Perform Clinical Procedures, First Edition. Matthew Stephenson, Joshua Shur and John Black.
© 2013 John Wiley & Sons, Ltd. Published 2013 by John Wiley & Sons, Ltd.

Procedure

Make sure you have the **correct patient**, for the **correct procedure**. Check for any **allergies**, and that you have confirmed the **indication;** excluded any **contraindications; explained** the procedure and taken **consent**. Now **wash your hands**!

Assemble all of your equipment on a trolley away from the patient. You will need everything in the equipment textbox.

Equipment you need

- Stockinette bandage
- Undercast padding (various widths)
- Plaster of Paris (various widths)
- Crepe bandage (various widths)
- Scissors
- Bucket of water (tepid temperature)
- A sling
- Adhesive tape
- Apron x 2
- Disposable gloves

Make sure your patient is **sitting comfortably** and has been prescribed adequate **analgesia**, particularly if a manipulation is required. Ideally the patient should be **seated** on a chair with the **arm supported** on an adjustable couch or equivalent armrest. This way you can move the limb up and down for the patient's own comfort not to mention the well-being of your own back. Inevitably, you are likely to make a mess given the nature of plastering. In addition to wearing a **plastic disposable apron** yourself, it's probably sensible to give one to the patient to wear too in order to save any spillage onto the patient's skin and clothing. Whilst the plaster readily washes out of clothing, direct contact with the skin can result in irritation. Check the patient doesn't have any rings on their fingers or a watch as these might affect circulation if the hand should swell following injury.

Depending on the patient's level of discomfort or amount of manipulation required, you may need another pair of hands to hold the wrist while you plaster, so try and get an **assistant**. Make sure the assistant tries to support the fracture site. For a non-displaced distal radial fracture, the patient's wrist should generally be in the **neutral position**.

The slab should be between **6 and 8 layers of plaster of Paris**, depending on whether you have an athlete or someone with less muscle bulk. The **width** of the slab will depend on the size of the patient's arm: 7.5 cm for a smaller arm or 10 cm for a larger one. Vary the thickness of your slab according to the type of patient. For example, for an elderly lady, who is not too active, 6 layers would suffice; for a young athlete, 7–8 layers would be ideal.

To **measure the length** of the slab hold one end at the coronoid process and the other to the metacarpophalangeal joints. Leave two finger breadth away from the coronoid process. This will allow for full movement of the fingers and elbow (important for swelling, checking neurovascular status and rehabilitation), so get trimming! Now you need to **cut a**

little half moon around where the plaster will oppose the first web space to allow for movement of the thumb.

Be sure to **round off the corners** of the slab, as when the plaster has hardened, these can potentially cause trauma to the soft tissues. **Repeat the measuring process** for the **stockinette** but leave slightly longer for folding back at either end – this protects the skin from the plaster edges. Have a bucket of water prepared. The **desired temperature is tepid** or body temperature.

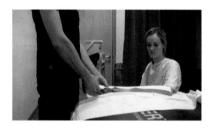
The upper limb is rested comfortably whilst the stockinette is measured

With your assistant supporting the patient's arm and wrist, **apply the stockinette** to the patient's arm – remember to leave it long! Take the **undercast padding** – a soft material sandwiched between the stockinette and plaster, and start two fingers away from the elbow crease progressing distally towards the fingers. **Overlap** the undercast padding by 50% over the previous turn as you go, finishing just before the metacarpal heads. If they have a prominent ulna styloid you might

want to either pop a little extra undercast padding on this or, if available, a spot of orthopaedic felt in order to maximise comfort.

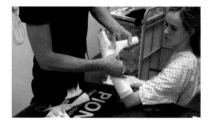
The undercast padding is applied

Holding the two ends of your previously measured plaster, gently **concertina** it up and submerge in the water for around 4 seconds. **Lift the plaster out**, lightly **squeeze** it over the bucket and **apply the slab** as per pre-plaster plan to the dorsal aspect of the patient's wrist and forearm. Smooth out the plaster (remember there is a broken arm in there, so don't go at it like a bull in a china shop!) making sure all the **creases and bubbles are gone. Start distally** from the central point, smoothing from side to side. **Mould** your plaster to the shape of the patient's anatomy, bearing in mind the whole purpose of this particular plaster is to **immobilise** the wrist. **Turn back the edges** of your stockinette, making sure the patient has full use of their fingers. You really want to be able to visualise the second palmar crease. Repeat the smoothing action proximally shaping it to fit the patient's forearm. Fold back the purposely excessive length of stockinette. **Check** that the patient's **elbow flexion is not limited**. However, they shouldn't be able to flex, extend, pronate or supinate the wrist. Apply your **crepe bandage**, starting at the distal end, working your way up proximally, again using 50–50 overlapping technique. For that professional look, finish the crepe bandage on the slab, not on the volar aspect, then fix the end with a short off cut of plaster or some 'inch pink' **adhesive tape** and smooth down.

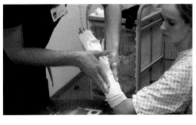

The moist plaster is moulded to the forearm

Wash off any plaster from the patient's skin, as it will make them itch, and remove their apron. It's vitally import to check that the patient has remained **neurovascularly intact**. Ask them to wiggle their fingers, check their sensation and capillary refill time. The plaster should be firm to the touch within 20 minutes but can take up to 24 hrs to fully dry. Supply the patient with a broad arm **sling** or collar and cuff for comfort and to reduce swelling. **Counsel** the patient with regards to the importance of elevation to prevent swelling, and the basic elements of cast care. Explain to them that they must return if the cast becomes too tight. Encourage them to open and close their fist in order to maintain adequate circulation and prevent stiffness. Don't forget to **book them into fracture clinic** for follow up and **document** everything you've done.

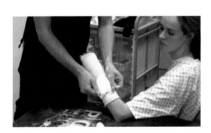

A small offcut of plaster is used to secure the crepe bandage in place

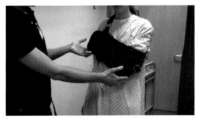

A sling must be worn to aid elevation and reduce swelling

8 Blood Culture

Video Time | 2 mins 35 s

Overview

In order to understand the purpose of a blood culture, it's important to appreciate that blood in the circulatory system of a healthy individual is theoretically deemed to be sterile. If bacteria has managed to enter the blood stream then the causative organism can sometimes be found from a sample of the individuals blood. This involves taking blood from the patient and transferring samples into artificial, bacteria friendly media, creating the optimal conditions for the bacteria's equivalent of an orgy: the blood culture. If a causative organism spreads to the blood stream, and the organisms are found on blood culture, then the patient is said to have a bacteraemia.

After culturing a bacteria, it's possible to test the organism's sensitivity to various antibiotics, to aid the clinician in selecting the most appropriate antimicrobial to treat the patient. Selecting an antibiotic that is specific for a pathogen, whilst leaving other non-pathogenic organisms alone, is important to minimise antibiotic resistance. It is important to culture your patient before starting empirical antibiotics as this can make later interpretation of blood cultures problematic. Once the culture has been sent to the lab, your empirical antibiotic therapy should cover most of the common pathogens whilst you await the culture results. Without the culture results, you are essentially treating your patient "blindly".

Bear in mind that the decision to prescribe antibiotics and the selection of antibiotic should be in adherence to trust protocol, and on the advice of a microbiologist if unsure.

How to Perform Clinical Procedures, First Edition. Matthew Stephenson, Joshua Shur and John Black.
© 2013 John Wiley & Sons, Ltd. Published 2013 by John Wiley & Sons, Ltd.

Sterility is of paramount importance when taking a culture. It's highly embarrassing when the hospital's microbiologist informs you that the sample you so carefully labelled has replicated nothing more than a zoo of the patient's natural skin flora. Most importantly, the results of the culture must be interpreted in the clinical context. If in doubt consult your seniors and your microbiology colleagues.

Indications	Contraindications	Complications
• Infection (known source) • Infection (unknown source) • Pyrexia of unknown origin • Raised inflammatory markers • Signs and symptoms of infection/sepsis	• End of life care pathway has been commenced	As of any venepuncture: • Bleeding • Haematoma • Phlebitis • Cellulitis • Septicaemia

Procedure

Make sure you have the **correct patient**, for the **correct procedure**. Check for any **allergies** (e.g. to the plaster you're going to put on at the end), and that you have confirmed the **indication;** excluded any **contraindications; explained** the procedure and taken **consent**. Now **wash your hands**!

Assemble all of your equipment on a trolley away from the patient. You will need everything in the equipment textbox. Cultures are best obtained from your patient during an **episode of pyrexia**. The pyrexia is assumed to reflect the systemic response to the increased concentration of any bacteraemia, and therefore increases your chances of a positive yield. However, blood cultures can still occasionally be

Equipment you need (on a sterile tray/trolley)

- Sterile pack containing:
  - Sterile gauze
  - Sterile field
  - Sterile gloves
- Tourniquet (disposable preferably)
- Butterfly needle
- Culture bottle collection device (e.g. modified Vacutainer)
- Alcohol wipes (for bottle tops)
- Anaerobic culture bottle (in date)
- Aerobic culture bottle (in date)
- Alcohol based skin preparation
- Adhesive tape
- Sharps bin

performed on apyrexial patients if the index of suspicion remains high.

Standard blood cultures should never be obtained from a venous cannula or other intravascular device (this includes central and arterial lines). This is because despite every effort, intravascular devices commonly become colonised with opportunistic organisms which will inevitably contaminate your sample, although if you suspect there might be a line infection, take cultures both through the line and peripherally. This will increase the chance of getting those bugs. However, if your index of suspicion is strong – the line should simply be removed straight away and a new one sited, along with cultures taken peripherally.

Wash your hands thoroughly and don your **gloves**. **Sterilise the skin** with an alcohol based wipe cleaning first over the intended puncture with an up and down/side-to-side motion, moving out in ever increasing circles. Leave the puncture site to dry.

With the puncture site dry, you can be relatively assured that your desired target skin is sterile. Apply the disposable **tourniquet** with enough tension to occlude the venous system. Assemble your collection apparatus by screwing the custom made Vacutainer collection device to the butterfly needle. Remember, your puncture site is now sterile and you should refrain from touching it again. A good tip is to palpate your vessel of choice before you clean the area. **Clean the tops** of your collection bottles with an alcohol based wipe and allow to dry. Warning your patient of an **impending sharp scratch**, desheath the butterfly, and bevel up,

advance the needle through the skin, into the vessel in exactly the same way you would for any venepuncture. Confirmation of successful venepuncture is defined by visualising **flashback** into the plastic tubing.

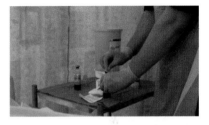

The bottle tops should be cleaned with an alcohol wipe to prevent contamination

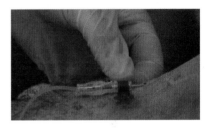

The butterfly needle is used here and flashback can be seen in the tubing

Once flashback is established, stabilise the positioning of the needle with your non-dominant hand. With the other, pick up the **anaerobic bottle first** and **slide the bottle** containing the culture medium into the Vacutainer. The bottles prepared for blood culture are vacuumed and are thus self-filling. As a result, blood should travel up the tube and begin to fill the bottle. Once you have collected the sample, pull the bottle out of the collection device, and repeat the same method, this time with the **aerobic bottle**. It's important to note that we are aiming for 3–5 mls of blood in each bottle. Too little, and you may miss your opportunity in detecting and replicating the culprit. Too much of the red stuff effectively acts as a diluent to the nutrients in the bottle which theoretically means the bacteria will have nothing to gnosh on. If you're also taking blood for other purposes from the Vacutainer, it's important to do the blood cultures first. This is because the other heparisined blood tubes are frequently contaminated with environmental non-fermenting organisms.

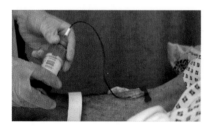

The blood culture bottle has been inserted into the Vacutainer and is filling by its own steam

After collecting the samples, **release the tourniquet**. Once the tourniquet is released, **withdraw the needle**, and apply direct pressure to the site. Dispose of the needle in the **sharps bin**. Finally apply a piece of **adhesive tape** to affix the gauze. **Thank** the patient and **dispose of your clinical waste** as appropriate.

Great! You have done the hard work, but equally as important is to ensure that the bottles are legibly and accurately **labelled**. This should include the patient's details, and also cite where the cultures were skilfully obtained. You will need to complete a **request form** as demonstrated in the video. Make sure that the details mirror the details on your bottles, and in addition give as much clinical information on the form as possible – it will be read by a human! Include all information about infection history and antibiotic use. Remember to sign and give a contact number or bleep. **Document** what you've done in the patient's notes.

Once you're happy with the samples, place them in a bag along with the request form. They are now ready to be sent to the lab and this should be done promptly in order to get them into the lab incubator quickly as many bugs die easily (especially pneumococcus). In the lab they will be analysed for **microscopy, culture and sensitivity** (M, C and S). This M, C and S means three different things. The first is a microscopic examination of the blood by the microbiology technician or even microbiologist and can provide a basic answer as to whether there's florid infection present, within an hour or two. Sometimes this is clinically crucial. The second is the culture result and a provisional result should be obtained within the first 24 hours as to the presence of bugs, but some take much longer to grow, for instance 5–7 days or longer.

The sensitivity of any cultured bugs is the third part and this is often available 48 hours after the test. A helpful microbiologist will usually contact you promptly (as long as you left legible contact details) if the samples yield any significant diagnosis which may alter the course of treatment for the patient. Otherwise, results are usually available through your hospital's pathology portal.

OSCE checklist

- Assembles equipment correctly
- Dons gloves
- Applies tourniquet
- Selects vein appropriately
- Cleans site
- Cleans culture bottle tops
- Warns about a 'sharp scratch'
- Inserts needle at appropriate angle
- Inserts anaerobic bottle
- Inserts aerobic bottle second
- Labels blood bottles
- Completes request forms
- Washes hands
- Thanks patient
- Disposes of sharps and waste
- Documents procedure
- Provides postprocedure advice

9 Blood Transfusion

Ruochen Li

Video Time | 3 mins 33 s

Overview

Blood unquestionably saves lives and improves the quality of life in an array of conditions. With approximately 3.34 million blood products transfused annually in the UK alone, it's big business. SHOT (serious hazards of transfusion, 2007) estimate that of the serious bulk of errors, 80% can be attributed to human error, with a staggering 42% of those errors occurring when collecting and checking blood prior to transfusion at the patient's bedside! Cumulative SHOT data from 1996/97 to 2011 show that almost 10 000 episodes of patient morbidity or mortality occurred and 159 deaths where transfusion reaction was either contributory or causal. Here cometh the warning ... Blood is arguably one of the most dangerous drugs you will ever prescribe/administer, so it's important to have a basic understanding of the exhaustive systematic checklist, how to safely administer the blood product, and an appreciation of the avoidable risk that recipients are exposed to of which in its extreme, can lead to serious morbidity and death. **Bedside checking is your last-chance saloon to prevent an error**.

So unsurprisingly, the UK blood service has produced national guidelines in *Handbook of Transfusion Medicine (2007)*. National guidelines such as these are responsible for informing local policy. This may vary from trust to trust, so familiarise yourself with trust guidelines and act accordingly. This chapter focuses on providing you with an overview of the bedside checking procedure and the physicality of giving blood through a giving set.

How to Perform Clinical Procedures, First Edition. Matthew Stephenson, Joshua Shur and John Black.
© 2013 John Wiley & Sons, Ltd. Published 2013 by John Wiley & Sons, Ltd.

Indications	Contraindications	Complications
• Severe anaemia (obviously!) (haemorrhage, trauma) • Chronic disorders (renal failure, malignancy) • Haemoglobinopathies (e.g. sickle cell disease, thalassaemia) • Marrow failure (aplastic anaemia, leukaemia) • Severe haemolysis (e.g. haemolytic disease of the newborn)	• Megaloblastic anaemia • Iron deficiency anaemia (transfusion in healthy individuals where use of oral iron could rectify a low Hb) • Caution with sickle cell patients	**Acute:** • Allergic reaction (mild to anaphylaxis) • Haemolytic reaction • Infective shock • Circulatory overload • Infection: HIV, hepatitis B&C, syphilis (rare in UK) • TRALI (Transfusion-Related Acute Lung Injury) **Delayed:** • Delayed haemolysis of transfused red blood cells • Transfusion associated graft Vs host disease • Posttransfusion purpura • Iron overload • Infection

Procedure

Before you get anywhere near the patient with a unit of blood, a valid group and save or crossmatch must be approved by the blood bank. This involves bleeding the patient and obtaining a pink-topped specimen sample (see Chapter 42: Venepuncture). The **patient identifiers must be clearly handwritten** on the bottle and the request form in your finest block capitals, obtained from the patient's wrist band with simultaneous verbal confirmation. Patient identification stickers should never be used. If the patient is unconscious on admission, they will be allocated a unique set of patient identifiers

which usually doesn't include their own name or date of birth. In any case, the principles remain the same: Use the unique identifiers to send for blood in a similar way. A blood bank request form is then completed. They are relatively self explanatory. **Be warned**: The details on the specimen bottle must correspond exactly to the details on the request form. If there are any discrepancies, the sample will be rejected and destroyed without any exceptions. You can also expect a hostile bleep from the bank informing you of your error! In an emergency, this can be extremely frustrating and delay treatment in an urgent situation. It's always worth asking a helpful colleague to check the sample and form before sending. It's an easy mistake to make, tired eyes make short work for the devil.

Blood products are stored in the blood bank. The most commonly transfused blood products are red cells. Other blood products transfused include fresh frozen plasma (FFP), cryoprecipitate and platelets. FFP is plasma with the full set of coagulation factors and is frozen immediately after collection. Blood product infusion should commence within 15–30 minutes of it leaving their preferential safe storage environment. Packed red blood cells should have been infused entirely within a maximum of 4 hours. If, for whatever reason there is any delay, the blood bank must be informed and the product returned. Prior to sending for the blood, check the reason for transfusion and that the blood has been prescribed correctly. Consider any special requirements, for example gamma irradiation if transfusing to immunocompromised patients. Additional drugs should never be added to the blood bag itself. It may precipitate a transfusion reaction which would be a catastrophe. Any additional medications required alongside the blood transfusion should be administered independently. Optimise bank-to-tranfusion time by checking the following: Does the patient have a patent cannula? Are there two trained members of staff available to administer the transfusion (for some trusts this is an absolute requirement)? Is the patient positioned correctly? Have a baseline set of observations been recorded? Clearly communicate your intentions with the nursing staff so that everything runs to clock work precision.

Blood is now usually dispensed via an electronic tracking system. This involves scanning a unique bar code on each individual unit as the blood leaves the bank. The blood is transported in a specially insulated box. On arrival to the ward, the blood is scanned a second time to confirm arrival. This allows precise tracking and provides an enhanced audit trail highlighting errors so that organisational training can occur.

Make sure you have the **correct patient**, for the **correct procedure**. Check for any **allergies** (e.g. to the plaster you're going to put on at the end), and that you have confirmed the **indication;** excluded any **contraindications; explained** the procedure and taken **consent**. Now **wash your hands**!

Assemble all of your equipment on a trolley away from the patient. You will need everything in the equipment textbox.

Equipment you need (on a sterile tray/trolley)

- A blood giving set
- Non-sterile gloves
- Apron
- Alcohol based wipe
- Saline flush
- Drip stand
- The unit of blood products for transfusion
- A patent cannula (sited in said patient)
- A verified group and save/crossmatch (done beforehand)

Position the patient (normally either sitting up or on a bed/trolley) so that they can be observed for any adverse reaction whilst the transfusion is taking place.

The blood will arrive within a box accompanied by a compatibility form and a compatibility label. The compatibility label consists of two components: A transfusion sticker and smaller stickers which are transferred to the patient's notes and drug chart. The unit of blood product will also be labeled. **Check that all patient identifiers correspond across all labels**.

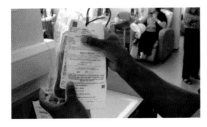

The blood bag which needs to be carefully checked

Begin by scanning the bar code with the electronic scanner (if your trust has such technology). As described earlier, blood is often electronically traced from origin to source to limit errors and enhance the audit trail. It allows organisational training to occur. A scanner is available on every ward. **Scan the bar code**, as if scanning a product in the supermarket. This communicates to the blood bank that the products have arrived to the ward as requested. You are now

ready to begin the arduous but crucial task of pre transfusion checking.

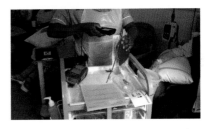

In this hospital a bar code scanning system is in operation

Wash your hands and **put on an apron** followed by a **pair of non-sterile gloves**. Remove the blood product from the box and visually inspect it. Look for:
- Pack integrity
- Presence of large clots
- Evidence of haemolysis in the plasma or at the interface between the red cells and the plasma
- The label on the blood product corresponds to the compatibility form and compatibility labels (as previously discussed) – unit number, product, blood group
- Expiry date

If there is an issue with any of the above points, the blood must not be infused and should be returned to the blood bank.

Checking must take place at the patient's bedside. Again, depending on trust policies two trained members of staff may be advised to oversee this process. Only ever check blood products one patient at a time: Multi-tasking is where many errors occur!

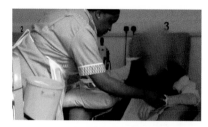

You must check the patient details correspond with the patient's wrist band

If you're interrupted during your checking proforma, you must start the process all over again irrespective of how time consuming the process can be. **Ask the patient** to tell you their full name and date of birth. **Ensure this information corresponds** to the patient's ID band and also with the information on the unit of blood and compatibility forms. **Check the unit number** on the blood itself corresponds with the unit number on the compatibility label. **Check the expiry date** on the unit of blood. Check that the blood has been prescribed correctly on the drug chart. Finally, ask the second trained member of staff to **begin their own identical checks**.

Once the checking is complete, a **routine baseline set of observations** should be performed and charted before the transfusion begins, including temperature, blood pressure, respiration rate and pulse rate. You're now ready to prime the giving set line.

A specific blood-giving set should be used for infusion of blood products. Blood-giving sets differ from regular giving

sets in that they have a double chamber and integral mesh filter. This is to prevent micro thrombi being administered to the patient. **Check the line** is within the manufacturer's use by date, and carefully remove it from the packaging. Generally speaking, electronic pumps are contraindicated in administration of blood, as they can damage the red blood cells, causing them to haemolyse.

Check the roller ball clamp on the line works, and **set it to the closed position**. This is really important or else you will end up with, quite literally, a blood bath. The blood unit has opposing plastic tabs protecting the site where you plunge the spike of the giving set into the blood unit – **pull the tabs** to expose the outlet port. This should be performed using a non touch technique (i.e. try not to touch the outlet port). **Remove the cap** from the giving set spike and, aseptically, **advance the spike** into the outlet port. The blood should fill the first chamber and part of the second chamber even with the roller ball clamp closed. Once the chambers have filled, **slowly open the roller ball clamp** and run the blood through the giving set all the way to the end ensuring that all air is expelled. Once the line is primed, **close the clamp** once more.

Take an alcohol based wipe and **clean the port** of the cannula, before **flushing** the line with 5–10 mls of normal saline. Aseptically **remove the cap** from the end of your giving set and **attach it to the cannula**. Secure the line to the patient with a bandage or some adhesive tape if necessary. Finally, **open your roller ball clamp**, and **slowly let the blood infuse**. Always begin any infusion slowly, as this gives you time to **observe the patient clinically** to check for any adverse reaction. Anaphylaxis is usually a rapid response, which can occur within the first few drops. The following offers a useful structured approach for monitoring for such reactions:

- Temperature, pulse and blood pressure before each unit
- Temperature and pulse 15 minutes after the start of each unit
- Temperature, pulse and blood pressure at the end of each unit
- Further observations should be at the discretion of each clinical area, dependent on, for example:
  - Unstable clinical condition
  - Level of consciousness
  - Inability to communicate adverse effects, for example if patient is a neonate or small child

If the patient displays any adverse signs, discontinue the infusion immediately.

When you're happy that the patient is tolerating the infusion, you can **increase the infusion rate**. This is usually between 2 and 4 hours per unit of blood depending on the cardiovascular status of the patient – nowadays it's relatively difficult to overload even an elderly patient with impaired cardiac function via a blood transfusion since the days of using whole blood are long gone, we are only using packed red cells. The use therefore of frusemide with blood transfusions should be rare. The blood should be infused within 4 hours as a maximum, as per transfusion guidelines.

The patient should be closely observed particularly within the first 15 minutes of commencing transfusion, as this is when a transfusion reaction is most likely to occur. Finally, adequate **documentation** is key. Make a note of the date, time and place that the transfusion was initiated, stating a clear indication. Include the type of blood product being transfused, the number of units to be transfused and the unit numbers in full. Ensure the **prescription is signed, timed and dated** along with a sticker from the transfusion label. The transfusion label, along with the compatibility form, should be filed in the patient's notes immediately following the transfusion.

- Uses correct blood giving set with filter
- Assembles equipment correctly
- Verbally confirms patient identifiers and cross checks
- Uses blood tracking system accurately
- Counsels patient with regards to transfusion reaction
- Understands transfusion rates and clinical checks required
- Inserts giving set spike into blood pouch
- Hangs blood unit up
- Cleans cannula connector
- Primes line appropriately
- Connects line appropriately
- Sets rate of infusion
- Transfers labels to drug chart
- Completes the necessary documentation accurately
- Washes hands
- Thanks patient

10 Bone Marrow Aspirate and Biopsy

Anita Sarma

Video Time | 4 mins 16 s

Overview

Bone marrow examination is one of the most important diagnostic tools available to a haematologist. The majority of bone marrow biopsies are still performed by haematology trainees and consultants. Some institutions, however, may have a designated bone marrow list for the haematology 'senior house officer' or bone marrow specialist nurse and as such we have included it in this book and DVD.

In an adult, haemopoeitically active bone marrow is restricted to cavities of the axial skeleton, with the most accessible sites being the pelvis and the sternum. The iliac crest is the only site at which both bone marrow aspiration and biopsy may be performed safely. The posterior iliac crest, located at the centre of the posterior superior iliac spine, is generally the preferred site, as it is considered the safest and least uncomfortable for the patient. Alternative sites include the anterior iliac crest and sternum and can be considered in patients who are immobile or obese. However, only experienced senior medical staff should perform sampling at these sites. This chapter describes bone marrow aspiration and biopsy from the posterior iliac crest.

Bone marrow examination is used in the diagnosis, staging and follow-up of haematological disease. In selected situations it may also be useful in patients with pyrexia of unknown origin (PUO) or to diagnose storage and infiltrative disorders. Specimens obtained through **bone marrow aspiration** are used to assess cellular morphology and to conduct specialised tests including flowcytometry for immunophenotyping, and cytogenetic and molecular genetic analysis.

How to Perform Clinical Procedures, First Edition. Matthew Stephenson, Joshua Shur and John Black.
© 2013 John Wiley & Sons, Ltd. Published 2013 by John Wiley & Sons, Ltd.

Indications	Contraindications	Complications

• Suspected haematological malignancy
  ◦ Myeloma
  ◦ Lymphoma
  ◦ Metastatic disease
  ◦ Atypical anaemia
• Bone marrow storage / infiltrative disorders / cellularity / architecture
• Bone marrow donation/ transplantation (matching process)
	• Consideration of coagulopathy, otherwise no absolute contraindications (if in doubt check the patient's clotting profile beforehand)	• Pain
		• Bleeding
		• Scar
		• Infection
		• Haematoma / bruising
		• Neurovascular injury

Bone marrow trephine biopsy is usually performed as an adjunct to bone marrow aspiration. It provides specific information about bone marrow architecture and cellularity, allowing assessment of the pattern and extent of infiltration in lymphoma, myeloma, metastatic disease and storage disorders.

Although there are no absolute contraindications to performing bone marrow aspiration and biopsy, the risk of procedure-related bleeding is more significant in patients with a coagulopathy. In such situations, consideration should be taken to reverse the coagulopathy as much as possible or delay the procedure until deemed safe. Furthermore, one should avoid obtaining a trephine biopsy if possible. Isolated thrombocytopenia on the other hand is not a contraindication for performing the procedure and prophylactic platelet transfusion is not usually recommended in these circumstances.

As with all procedures, preparation is the key to a straightforward and safe experience for both patient and operator. It is useful to speak to the laboratory or the person requesting the investigation before the procedure to determine which tests are required and which specimen bottles should be used. Often, guidance may differ depending on which trust you work for, so familiarise yourself with the local policy beforehand.

Procedure

It's preferable to have an assistant when performing bone marrow aspiration and biopsy to monitor and provide additional reassurance to the patient, as well as assisting the operator with preparing specimens. If sedation of any kind is administered a trained nurse must attend to the patient throughout the entire procedure. Supplemental oxygen must be provided and routine observations must be monitored continuously in order to maintain patient safety.

Make sure you have the **correct patient**, for the **correct procedure**. Check for any **allergies**, and that you have confirmed the **indication;** excluded any **contraindications; explained** the procedure and taken **consent**. Now **wash your hands**!

Assemble all of your equipment on a sterile trolley away from the patient. You will need everything in the equipment textbox.

Remember that bone marrow aspiration and biopsy is a daunting and uncomfortable procedure for the patient. Creating a calm and reassuring environment is just as important as providing adequate local anaesthesia and sedation in making this procedure as tolerable as

possible. The pain experienced by patients undergoing bone marrow aspiration and biopsy with local anaesthesia is typically minimal to moderate. However, some individuals with significant anxiety or those who have undergone multiple prior procedures may have a heightened sense of pain. Safe conscious sedation with benzodiazepines or inhaled nitrous oxide can be used to reduce anxiety and ameliorate pain. In order for the premedication to have its full effect the operator needs to ensure that it's administered quickly prior to the start of the procedure.

Position the patient in the **lateral decubitus** position with the back comfortably flexed and the knees drawn towards the chest, sometimes also referred to as the foetal position. Alternatively, the patient may be placed in the prone position.

It's helpful to **locate the posterior iliac spine** before creating the sterile field. The usual site for aspiration and biopsy is located three fingerbreadths from the midline and two fingerbreadths inferior to the iliac crest. It may be helpful

Equipment you need (on a sterile tray/trolley)

- Sterile gloves and gown
- Alcohol/chlorhexidine swabs
- Sterile gauze
- Sterile dressing
- Sterile drape
- Green needle (25G) x 2
- Blue needle (23G) x 2
- Orange needle (21G) x 2
- 2 ml syringe
- 10 ml syringe x 2
- Local anaesthesia/sedation (caution if required)
- Bone marrow aspirate/trephine needle (usually prepacked as one entity)
- Glass slides (frost ended)
- Slide holder
- Pencil (for labelling)
- Sample bottles containing appropriate mediums
- Container with formalin solution (for trephine cut)

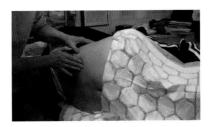

Palpating the posterior iliac spine to identify the biopsy site to make a light mark with the cap of a pen on the skin overlying the site.

Using an aseptic technique, **clean the skin** with antiseptic and drape as appropriate. **Infiltrate** the skin, subcutaneous tissue and periosteum with **local anaesthetic**. Warn the patient that the local anaesthetic will sting a little and that this can be especially uncomfortable when anaesthetising the periosteum, as it is extremely sensitive. It is crucial that an adequate area of the periosteum is infiltrated with local anaesthetic to allow for an aspirate and biopsy to be performed through the same skin needle tract, but at different sites on the iliac crest approximately 1 cm apart. Leave sufficient time for the anaesthetic to take effect. Before proceeding further, gently probe the surrounding periosteum with the needle to ensure no sensitive areas remain.

Part 1: Bone marrow aspiration

After obtaining an aspirate, the samples will need to be spread onto slides for later examination. It's therefore good practice to prepare your slides before starting. Try to prepare a minimum of 6 beforehand, but more rather than less is preferable.

Aspiration needles have an adjustable guard, required when performing a sternal puncture. This can be removed when aspirating from the iliac crest to provide greater needle length. It may be found that in very obese patients the average aspirate needle is not long enough to reach the bone. In such cases special

long aspirate needles may be available, or alternatively a longer trephine needle can be used.

If aspirate and biopsy are performed in sequence, an incision to the skin at the marked site is not necessary. It may be required to make a 3 mm incision first, when only a biopsy is needed, or if the calibre of the biopsy needle is particularly large, to facilitate entry.

It's important to understand that bone marrow aspiration and biopsy requires a certain sensibility, control and gentle pressure. Force or significant strength is hardly ever required. **Hold the needle** with the proximal end in palm and the index finger against the shaft near the tip. This stabilises the needle and allows for better control.

Insert the needle perpendicular to skin at the marked site, **advancing the needle** carefully to the periosteum. Before pushing further, ensure a secure position on the flat area of the iliac crest. Place the other hand on the patient's hip to improve stability and awareness of the position and direction of the needle.

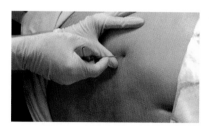

Inserting the needle before taking the bone marrow aspirate

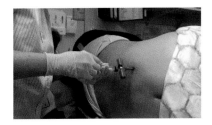

Taking the aspirate

Pointing the needle toward the anterior superior iliac spine, apply gentle pressure and **advance the needle through the periosteum**, by rotating the needle in a back and forth motion. When entering the marrow cavity a 'give' or a change in resistance should be felt. The patient may experience discomfort at this point or on removing the stylette. Warn the patient of this possible discomfort.

Advance the needle no more than 1 cm beyond the periosteum. The needle should be securely anchored in the bone. **Remove the stylette** and attach the 2 ml syringe. Alert the patient to possible brief suction pain before you pull the plunger. Typically, aspiration is the most

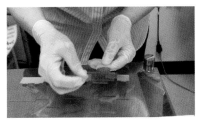

Preparing the slides of the bone marrow aspirate with a 'squash'

uncomfortable stage of the procedure (providing you have given adequate local anaesthesia to the periosteum).

Aspirate no more than 0.25–0.5 ml of concentrated aspirate and exchange the 2 ml syringe with a larger 10 or 20 ml syringe, ready for further aspiration. The concentrated aspirate in the 2 ml syringe should be **spread on the prelaid out slides** immediately to reduce the risk of clotting. The presence of bony particles or spicules may be immediately apparent on initial aspiration or at least as the first slide is spread. If the sample is adequate numerous granular irregularities in the aspirate will be seen. **Apply a small drop of aspirate** on to each slide in the centre line approximately one cm beyond the frosted end of the slide. Place another slide or spreader just in front of the drop at a 30° angle to the base slide and pull it back, allowing the drop to spread along the edge of the spreader. Then in one smooth swift motion, spread the aspirate forward along the slide, without lifting the spreader until the aspirate is fully spread. The size of the drop determines the length of the spread, ideally not exceeding 3 cm and finishing about 1 cm before the end of the slide. If performed correctly there should be a nice particle-rich feathered end. Essentially you are aiming to produce a monolayer of cells. This will need some practice, but will be consistently achieved with time. Time should also be spent practising spreading towards and away from the frosted end, as depending on local practice either direction may be preferred.

If the aspirate sample is very haemodilute there are concentration techniques that can be used to improve the quality of the sample. This may involve placing a large drop of aspirate on to one end of a slide, and aspirating off the excess liquid with a plastic pipette to reveal the particles, which can then be spread along the slide. There are other concentration techniques, which, for the inexperienced practitioner can be a little messy.

Once the slides are spread, **complete the aspiration process** by obtaining sufficient bone marrow to add to the various specimen bottles containing either preservative free heparin or EDTA. These can then be processed for further testing.

Occasionally no particles are obtained, despite easily aspirating bone marrow blood. This may either be due to being too shallow, or occasionally too deep within the bone. In this case, replace the stylette and gently manoeuvre the needle further out, or push it a little deeper. If there are still no particles on aspiration, attempt to reinsert the needle into the marrow cavity further along the iliac crest. If the aspirate is still aparticulate, this is known as a 'dry tap', which can be the result of fibrosis or a heavily infiltrated bone marrow. In such a situation a touch preparation using the cylinder from the core biopsy can be used instead. This is done by rolling the trephine specimen down a fresh slide, which leaves particles behind that can be stained and assessed for cellular morphology.

Once sufficient aspirate has been collected, and slides have been prepared, the **aspirate needle may be removed**, whereupon **gentle pressure** with some gauze should be applied until the oozing (if any) has stopped.

Part 2: Bone marrow biopsy

Before proceeding with the **bone marrow biopsy**, ensure that local anaesthesia to skin and periosteum is still adequate. Using a needle and syringe containing the local anaesthetic, probe the skin and periosteum and **inject more anaesthetic** if needed.

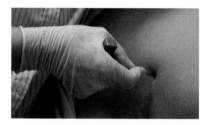

Bone marrow needle in place just prior to taking the bone marrow biopsy

Holding the trephine needle like the aspirate needle, **introduce it into the previous puncture site**. **Advance it** to the periosteum and move it along the iliac crest about 1 cm from the aspirate puncture site. Applying controlled pressure **penetrate the periosteum**. Ensure the needle is firmly lodged in the cortical bone before removing the stylette. **Advance the cutting needle** a further 2 cm, coring out the biopsy from the surrounding bone marrow tissue. **Warn the patient** that they may feel a deep-seated dragging sensation down the leg lasting a few seconds. To dislodge the core biopsy, **twist the needle 360°** in both directions several times, and advance the needle a few mm further before removing the biopsy needle. This is thought to reduce the risk of losing the cylinder in the biopsy tract on withdrawal of the needle. Some of the newer biopsy needles systems come with forceps-like extraction cannulas, which are inserted into the cutting needle, before removing it. This makes for a very neat biopsy which can then be pushed out of the cannula using the obturator probe.

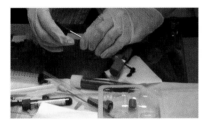

Extracting the core biopsy from the needle

Immediately after removing the biopsy needle place some sterile gauze and a sterile dressing over the wound and **apply pressure** for several minutes until haemostasis is achieved. Ask the patient to lie supine to apply indirect pressure on the biopsy site for about 10–15 minutes.

Additional care needs to be taken when obtaining trephine biopsy in patients with severe thrombocytopenia. Apply firm manual pressure to the biopsy site for about five minutes until primary haemostasis is achieved.

Now **extract the core biopsy from the needle**, by placing the guard on the distal end of the needle and pushing the cylinder out either on to a clean slide to make a touch preparation, or directly into a specimen pot containing formalin. The biopsy should be between 1.5 and 2.5 cm in length, and must be inspected for the lack of excessive cortical bone or cartilage, before completing the procedure.

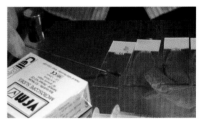

Rolling the biopsy over the slide

Label the slides with a pencil on the frosted end of the slide with the patient's name, hospital number and the date of the procedure. Either hand label or attach the appropriate label to each of your specimen pots and hand deliver the specimen to the laboratory.

Ensure the **patient is comfortable** and that there is no delayed or prolonged bleeding from the biopsy site. Explain to the patient that there may be a dull ache for a day, which can be relieved by **simple analgesia** such as paracetamol. Instruct the patient to keep the dressing dry for 24 hours and to leave the dressing on until the puncture site is scabbed over. Encourage the patient to avoid any strenuous activity for 24 hours to avoid delayed bleeding or pain. Although procedure-associated complications are rare it must be reiterated to the patient that they should seek medical attention if they experience prolonged pain, erythema, swelling indicative of infection or late bleeding.

Finally, **document the procedure** clearly in the notes. The site of the procedure should be stated, along with how much local anaesthetic was needed and type and amount of sedation if appropriate. Make a comment about the consistency of the bone and the quality of the aspirate with a specific mention of how particulate the sample was. State how many slides were made and how many samples were taken for what tests. Regarding the trephine biopsy, comment on the quality and length of the specimen. The number of attempts that were required to obtain each specimen should also be documented. Document any complications during the procedure, such as excessive pain, abnormal observations or prolonged or excessive bleeding.

OSCE checklist

- Assembles equipment correctly
- Positions patient correctly
- Identifies biopsy site
- Prepares slides
- Cleans site
- Administers local anaesthetic
- Removes guard
- Advances successfully through cortex
- Removes introducer
- Aspirates sample
- Removes needle
- Correctly prepares slides
- Advances needle through cortex
- Removes introducer
- Turns needle
- Removes needle
- Places guard and removes sample successfully
- Prepares slides with sample
- Places dressing
- Labels samples
- Stores slides
- Documents procedure in clinical notes
- Washes hands
- Thanks patient

11 Capillary Glucose Measurement

Video Time | 1 min 45 s

Overview

With an ever-increasing incidence of obesity, coupled with increased life expectancy, healthcare professionals face the monumental task of dealing with the detrimental effects of diabetes-related multi-system disease in an ageing population. As one of the major modifiable cardiovascular risk factors, it's important that we get it right with optimal therapeutic management and empowering the patient to take a shared responsibility through adequate education. Despite medical research and advancing insight into the causes and complications, the significance of managing one common theme is continually reiterated: The importance of glucose monitoring and tight glycaemic control remains essential in primary and secondary disease prevention.

Patients with diabetes are renowned for their fragility and poor reserve, particularly as they age. Not only are they prone to the chronic effects of poor glycaemic control, they frequently present in the acute setting with hyper or hypoglycaemic episodes. This is normally secondary to an acute concurrent illness, such as infection or dehydration, leading to diabetic ketoacidosis or hyperosmolar non-ketoacidosis. Suboptimal insulin regimes/other glucose lowering therapies falling short of the mark can spell trouble. Remember, diabetes management is dynamic, as can be the patient's glycaemia and glycaemic control. This highlights the importance of glucose monitoring, both as an inpatient and by the patient themselves in the community setting.

As a clinician it's important to appreciate the sometimes subtle, insidious onset of diabetes, and thus the importance of performing a glucose measurement as part of a primary survey in the acutely unwell or unconscious patient in the emergency

How to Perform Clinical Procedures, First Edition. Matthew Stephenson, Joshua Shur and John Black.
© 2013 John Wiley & Sons, Ltd. Published 2013 by John Wiley & Sons, Ltd.

setting should not be underestimated. Remember, if missed, the consequences can be catastrophic, and you will kick yourself forever and a day at your oversight when lamenting on the simplicity of this crucial, yet simple procedure.

Nowadays, we tend to measure blood glucose with either a venous blood sample (which has to be sent to the lab), or with a bedside capillary (as the blood is drawn from the capillary bed of the finger) blood glucose measurement. A multitude of 'bedside' or Point Of Care Testing (POCT) devices exist nowadays that can measure capillary blood glucose in a few seconds. The capillary glucose measurement is a very good surrogate marker for the 'blood' glucose.

Colloquially you will know it as the **BM**. What does BM stand for? Boehringer Manheim, obviously (this was the name of the company that originally made the test strips, but BM is now essentially synonymous with capillary glucose measurement).

Since POCT machines were introduced there have been errors associated with their use. This has often been down to staff not understanding their machine's limitations and when its use is inappropriate. For that reason it's absolutely crucial that you properly familiarise yourself with the one at your trust, including reading its operating manual. The main situations which may give a false result using a capillary BM machine are listed below, **however these may vary between machines** (taken from the MHRA safety notice Extra Laboratory Use of Blood Glucose Meters and Test Strips: Contraindications, Training and Advice to the Users. MDA SN 9616 June 1996).

Indications	Contraindications	Complications
• Diabetic patients (hospital and community) • Acute illness • Chronic diseases • Acute presentations to hospital • The unconscious patient • Screening in specific diseases	• Impairment in peripheral circulation, i.e. shock may cause inaccurate results • Haematocrit values above 55% may cause inaccurate results in glucose levels above 11 mmol/L • IV infusion of ascorbic acid • Preeclampsia • Some dialysis treatments • Hyperlipidaemia >13 mmol/L • Certain maltose/galactose treatments	• Bleeding (very rare) • Infection (very rare) • False/positive results (very rare)

Procedure

A capillary glucose measurement is performed by purposely inflicting a small amount of trauma to the skin, enough to draw blood. The known diabetic will have undoubtedly experienced this procedure before umpteen times and will often be completely proficient at doing it on themselves. However, there is a first time for everything, and as with any procedure, your intentions should be explained to the patient particularly if they are a capillary glucose measurement virgin.

Don't be alarmed by the amount of variation of capillary glucose monitoring kits and sensors out there. They all work universally on variations of a theme. If in doubt, take the time to familiarise yourself with the kits supplied by your trust.

Often in the hospital setting, the glucose measurement is electronically logged and therefore will require you to 'scan' the patient's notes (usually a bar code) or at worst input the patient's details manually as prompted. A friendly nurse will know how and if bribed with confectionary, will demonstrate this process effortlessly.

Before you take the machine to the bedside make sure the strips are in date and that the machine has been properly calibrated and has sufficient batteries. Often the machine will need to be recalibrated for each new set of test strips and set of batteries. Check the manufacturer's guidelines.

Make sure you have the **correct patient**, for the **correct procedure**.

Check for any **allergies**, and that you have confirmed the **indication;** excluded any **contraindications; explained** the procedure and taken **consent**. Now **wash your hands!**

Assemble all of your equipment on a trolley away from the patient. You will need everything in the equipment textbox and this is usually housed altogether on a designated **capillary glucose monitoring trolley**.

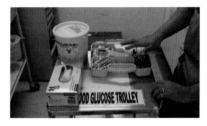

The capillary glucose measurement trolley with all the equipment ready

Equipment you need (on a sterile tray/trolley)

- Capillary glucose monitor
- Test strips
- Spring loaded needle 'lancet'
- Gloves
- Alcohol based wipes
- Gauze
- Plaster (occasionally)

Classically, the **ring or little finger** is used to obtain your sample, as the index finger when opposed to the thumb constitutes the pincer grip and can be painful. The lateral aspect of the finger is your target, just distal to the distal interphalangeal joint of the finger. Sites should be rotated to reduce the effects of trauma from repeated sampling.

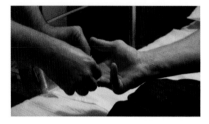

The lateral side of the finger is cleaned to wipe off any skin contaminants.

Wash your hands and put on a pair of **non-sterile gloves**. Carefully **tear the foil top** off the wrapping containing the chemically active disposable '**test strip**' (although bear in mind that these sticks don't always come foil-packed and may come in pots, for instance). The tear mark is usually clearly indicated and perforated for ease of tear. This exposes the end of the test strip which is inserted into the monitoring system. **Insert the test strip into the machine**, and make sure the machine is turned on and fully functional.

Next, **arm your lancet**. The lancet used to pierce the skin is usually spring loaded, and activated by twisting the top, or in some cases drawing back on the lever. Again, this can vary dependent on the trust you work in and may take a little familiarisation. The needle is usually deployed by pressing the trigger on the side, so be careful if you have it in your hand or you may experience an unexpected prick yourself.

Clean the skin, particularly if they have been noshing down sugared ring doughnuts (which hopefully they haven't) as this may contaminate the blood sample giving you a falsely high glucose reading. Tentatively **remove the foil** from the collection end, taking care not to touch it (this may also be a source of contamination).

Warning the patient of an **impending scratch**, **deploy the needle**. As it's spring loaded, it will penetrate to a set depth only. **Discard of your sharp** immediately in a sharps bin. **Encourage bleeding from** the site of trauma by gently squeezing the finger, until a droplet of blood is achieved. Lower the test strip to the sample. The blood will draw up onto the test strip automatically and will confirm when an adequate sample has been yielded electronically. Dependent on the monitoring system, the test usually takes around 20–30 seconds to produce a result. Whilst the test is running, **wipe up any excess blood** with the gauze on your trolley and apply a plaster if necessary/requested by the patient. Thank the patient for their sample and return the trolley so you don't get in trouble with Sister.

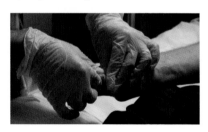

Squeeze out a drop of blood from the puncture site.

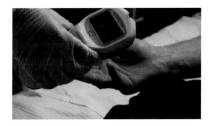

The glucose stick which is fixed into the machine is dipped into the spot of blood, and the timer begins.

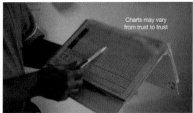

Make sure you record your result in the observations folder.

Chart your result on the relevant table in the patient's notes, with the time and date the test was performed. Make a note of any trends. If the result warrants urgent action, do it now! A glucose for instance of 1.2 mmol/l in an obtunded patient – the test is right and doesn't need repeating, the patient needs sugar stat! **Dispose of the used test strip** in the clinical waste bin and **wash your hands**.

12 Cardioversion

John Gomes

Video Time | 4 mins 44 s

Overview

Direct current cardioversion (DCCV) involves the use of **electric current** to convert an abnormal heart rhythm to sinus rhythm. This is done for five types of arrhythmia: atrial fibrillation (AF) (either emergency or elective), atrial flutter, ventricular tachycardia (VT), ventricular fibrillation (VF) or supraventricular tachycardia refractory to pharmacological cardioversion. **It's the quickest and most effective way of restoring sinus rhythm**. However, a year later, 50% of patients with AF who have been successfully cardioverted will have returned to AF.

Atrial fibrillation or atrial flutter are the most common indications for DC cardioversion and are discussed together as similar considerations apply to both. The main risk of cardioversion is that a **stroke** can be caused by restoring sinus rhythm. This is due to **stasis** of blood in the **left atrial appendage** during AF and this thrombus can be dislodged once the atria start contracting normally after sinus rhythm has been restored. The risk of stroke becomes significant **after 48 hours** in AF. If patients are significantly haemodynamically compromised (e.g. pulmonary oedema, hypotension, myocardial ischaemia), then the **risks** of remaining in atrial fibrillation are likely to **outweigh** the risk of stroke and urgent DC cardioversion should be considered. However, bear in mind that patients with long-standing AF are **unlikely** to revert to sinus rhythm following cardioversion.

Patients who are in AF for <48 hours can be cardioverted **safely**, if pharmacological treatments fail or they do not spontaneously cardiovert. They should still be **anticoagulated** with full dose low molecular weight heparin (LMWH) initially.

How to Perform Clinical Procedures, First Edition. Matthew Stephenson, Joshua Shur and John Black.
© 2013 John Wiley & Sons, Ltd. Published 2013 by John Wiley & Sons, Ltd.

Patients who are haemodynamically stable but have been in AF for >48 hours (or uncertain duration), will need formal anticoagulation with **warfarin**. NICE recommends anticoagulation for at least three weeks, but in practice most clinicians will anticoagulate for about **four weeks** prior to cardioversion. This can be confirmed with serial INRs in the weeks leading up to the procedure. If facilities are available, patients who are not anticoagulated can have a **transoesophageal echo** (TOE) prior to the procedure to check the atria and left atrial appendage for thrombus. If no thrombus can be identified in the heart, they can be cardioverted.

Patients in SVT or VT should have DC cardioversion as soon as possible. If they are haemodynamically stable, you have time to wait for an anaesthetist to sedate the patient before shocking them. Clearly, for a patient in ventricular fibrillation, you will **follow the ALS algorithm** and deliver an unsynchronised shock as soon as possible.

Indications	Contraindications	Complications
• Restoration of sinus rhythm	• Relative: • Inadequate anticoagulation and no TOE available (if AF > 48 hrs duration) • Hypokalaemia • Digoxin toxicity	• Stroke • Skin burns • Ventricular arrhythmia (VT/VF) • Asystole requiring pacing • Damage to pacemaker system

Procedure

Make sure you have the **correct patient**, for the **correct procedure**. Check for any **allergies**, and that you have confirmed the **indication;** excluded any **contraindications; explained** the procedure and taken **consent**. This is usually a signed consent form for elective patients. They will also need to see the anaesthetist and be kept **nil by mouth** for at least 4 hours prior to the procedure.

A 12 lead ECG should be performed for elective patients to check they still

Equipment you need

- Defibrillator
- Pads
- IV cannula and saline flush
- Equipment for induction and monitoring of general anaesthesia, including blood pressure and SO$_2$ monitoring
- Full resuscitation equipment

are in AF. Next, check the patient is adequately **anticoagulated** (if it's being done for AF). They should have a record of their INRs taken weekly for at least 3–4 weeks prior to the procedure and they should all be in the therapeutic range. If they have been in AF for <48 hours, they should have had LMWH.

Check recent **U&E** results to ensure **K$^+$ ≥3.5** and check their digoxin level if they are on high dose digoxin or in the presence of renal impairment. DCCV is much less likely to succeed if the patient is relatively hypokalaemic, and if digoxin levels are high, they are more susceptible to ventricular arrhythmia. Also, check that thyroid function tests have been performed and that they are in the normal range.

You now need to gain IV access and apply the defibrillation pads. Pad placement can either be **anteriorposterior** or **anterolateral** (as demonstrated in the video).

The pads should then be **connected to the defibrillator** and the 3 ECG leads from the machine also attached to the patient. Different defibrillator manufacturers have different ways of setting up their machines, and you should familiarise yourself with the device you will be using beforehand. Set the defibrillator to **manual mode** (not AED) and display a **lead II ECG** from the leads. This will usually give you a clear QRS complex with tall R waves – if not, change to a different lead configuration (e.g. lead I or III). You can also use the **gain setting** on the machine to give you a better trace.

General anaesthesia is then commenced by the anaesthetist with full monitoring. Once the patient is adequately sedated, the '**synchronise**' button on

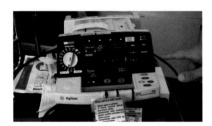

Defibrillator with SYNC displayed

Anteroposterior pad placement (i.e. one pad next to the left sternal edge over the heart and the other one on the patient's back in line with the first one) has been shown to have a better success rate than anterolateral pad placement. Pads should be kept away from pacemakers.

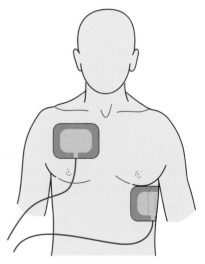

Diagram demonstrating Anterolateral pad placement

the defibrillator should be pressed. You should see arrows or other markers on the R waves on the defibrillator display. Make sure no markers appear on the T waves – change the lead configuration if they do. This ensures the shock is delivered on the **R wave** and not the T wave, which could lead to VT or VF.

Charge the defibrillator using your own hospital guidelines for the starting energy. For a biphasic defibrillator (the most common type), this is usually **100 J** for atrial flutter (it's more susceptible to electrical cardioversion) and **150 J** for atrial fibrillation and ventricular tachycardia. Switch the defibrillator printer on to get a printout for the notes.

Give a **warning** to make sure others in the room (and you!) are standing away from the bed and that the oxygen mask has been **removed**. You can now **press the button** to deliver the shock. There may be a slight delay in shock delivery as the machine ensures the shock is synchronised to the R wave. Put the oxygen mask back on the patient and **check the rhythm**. It's quite common for patients to be asystolic or in a slow junctional rhythm for a couple of seconds postprocedure. If it persists for any longer than this, **external temporary pacing or inotropes** may be required.

If the patient is now in sinus rhythm, check the blood pressure and the anaesthetist will wake the patient up.

If they are still in AF or VT, make sure the defibrillator is still synchronised to the R wave and charge again at 200 J this time and deliver the shock. If this isn't successful, a **third** shock can be attempted. A **maximum** of three shocks should be delivered.

A brief summary of the procedure should be **documented** in the notes and the rhythm strips attached.

The patient should be **monitored** for about 2 hours in a recovery ward following the procedure. If the patient has a pacemaker, the pacemaker should be **checked** afterwards. Warfarin should be continued in all patients until their next clinic appointment, even if DCCV is successful. Take **senior advice** about continuing other antiarrhythmic medication.

OSCE checklist

- Turns machine on
- Selects appropriate starting energy
- Obtains rhythm by selecting lead
- Ensures SYNC is selected
- Attaches appropriate monitoring
- Positions patient correctly
- Places pads correctly
- Induces general anaesthesia
- Charges machine
- Ensures it is safe to shock
- Delivers shock correctly
- Confirms sinus rhythm
- Documents procedure in notes

13 Central Venous Line

Reshma Woograsingh and Christopher Parnell

Video Time | 8 mins 50 s

Overview

Central venous access is a core skill for anaesthetists, critical care doctors and physicians alike. It allows **measurements of Central Venous Pressure** (CVP) to be made and also allows a **route of administration** for certain drugs which can't be given by the peripheral route without the risk of vein irritation, for example vaso-pressors such as noradrenaline, inotropes such as adrenaline and medications such as amiodarone and total parenteral nutrition.

Many centres provide an anaesthetic-led service for provision of central venous access which necessitates a clean environment, usually in an anaesthetic room, with ultrasound available as per **NICE guideline TA49**. The days of shoving a central line into random patients on dirty general medical wards with minimal attention to sterility are long gone. The best opportunities as an F1/F2 to learn to put in central lines therefore are to get friendly with the anaesthetic team. Not many days go by when the CEPOD list doesn't have a central line booked on it, and most anaesthetists are more than keen to teach juniors how to put them in. In fact in some hospitals, they will have the added hidden agenda that if they can teach you how to do it, then you can put all your own central lines in your own patients in future – many anaesthetists will tell you they're busy enough without also being the sole source of central lines for inpatients.

How to Perform Clinical Procedures, First Edition. Matthew Stephenson, Joshua Shur and John Black.
© 2013 John Wiley & Sons, Ltd. Published 2013 by John Wiley & Sons, Ltd.

Indications	Contraindications	Complications
• Very poor peripheral access requiring IV medications or fluid • CVP monitoring in the context of complex fluid balance and resuscitation • In conjunction with inotropes and vasopressors in HDU/ITU • Haemofiltration • Access for pulmonary artery catheters • Access for temporary pacing wires	• Localised infection over the intended site (absolute) • Bleeding diathesis • Vein for intended puncture is known to be occluded	• Localised bleeding and haeamatoma • Pneumothorax (the risk increases the lower the insertion site) • Haemothorax • Catheter related blood stream infection • Line thrombosis (resulting in occlusion) • Arrhythmias • Arterial puncture/perforation • Malposition of line • Air embolism (rare) • Neurological: brachial plexus injury, Horner's syndrome • Chylothorax

Sites of central venous access

These are the internal jugular, subclavian and femoral veins on either side. Each site has its own benefits and disadvantages: the choice will be governed by **patient factors** such as positioning the patient safely and easily, the ease of access in each patient – for example, the presence of known thrombosis or history of recent cannulation. The **indication** will also dictate the site of insertion: for instance, femoral access may be preferred for insertion of temporary pacing wires. In addition, the potential **complications** at each site may determine where the line is inserted as well as the individual's experience, not to mention competence!

An assessment of patency of the intended vessel should be made in terms of history of previous difficult attempts at cannulation and also previous surgical procedures which may make the whole exercise all the more tricky. A cursory look with the ultrasound before you start may also help identify potential problems. If the patient has an existing pneumothorax, it's probably a good idea to insert the line on that side so as to avoid the same complication arising on the other side.

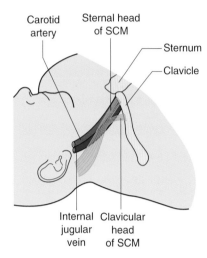

Carotid artery
Sternal head of SCM
Sternum
Clavicle
Internal jugular vein
Clavicular head of SCM

The route of the internal jugular vein in the neck, just lateral to the carotid artery and beneath the sternocleidomastoid

Procedure

Make sure you have the **correct patient**, for the **correct procedure**. Check for any **allergies**, and that you have confirmed the **indication;** excluded any **contraindications; explained** the procedure and taken **consent** which should be in the written form.

A **place of safety** to insert the line is paramount and will require availability of monitoring including continuous **ECG**, non-invasive **BP** and **SpO2** as a minimum. An **assistant** will also need to be available to help as well as an **ultrasound machine**. An **aseptic technique is mandatory** and **full surgical attire is compulsory**: gloves, gown, hat and mask. This is to avoid the risk of catheter related bloodstream infections.

Assemble all of your equipment on a sterile trolley away from the patient. It's important to use the correct type of central line for the patient. These vary in the number of lumens (between 3 and 5) and also on the length (between 15 and 20 cm). Ideally, the shorter line is used for right sighted internal jugular cannulation and the longer lines used for left sided and femoral access to avoid the tip ending up all the way into the right atrium.

Equipment you need (on a sterile tray/trolley)

- Sterile gauze
- The central line pack which contains:
  - Central line
  - Guidewire
  - Dilator
  - Needle introducer and/or cannula
  - 3-way taps or hubs for each lumen
- Cleaning solution, e.g. Betadine
- 5 ml syringe to attach needle introducer/ cannula
- 10 ml syringe for local anaesthetic
- 10 ml of local anaesthetic, e.g. lidocaine
- 20 ml syringe for normal saline
- Green (21G) needle
- Blue (23G) needle
- Sterile drapes
- Ultrasound probe cover
- Coupling media (gel for the ultrasound probe)
- A pot for saline
- Blade
- A dressing to secure to the skin
- Optional: suture
- Transparent, bio-occlusive dressing

The patient is **positioned appropriately** with the neck fully exposed and connected to the **monitoring**, **supine** with the **head turned to the contralateral side** so as to expose the anatomy more clearly. Often a **Trendelenburg** position (head end down) will aid filling of the vessel and therefore increase the size of the target and reduce the incidence of the dangerous complication of air embolism.

Once you have **scrubbed**, **prepare your equipment** in a logical order on your trolley so you can proceed in a timely fashion. One good way to set it out is with the needle, wire, dilator and cannula in that order. **Flushing the central line with saline** before you start is very important to avoid the small but significant risk of air embolism and also to check the lumens are flushing OK.

Clean the area with Betadine. Apply the **sterile drape** and using the ultrasound, **anaesthetise the intended area** with lidocaine 1% to cover the puncture site and sutures as well.

In the video you can see the probe being used to locate the vein before scrubbing up to identify its position and check that it's patent. It's then not used any further in the procedure. You can do it this way if you have plenty of experience, however alternatively you use the probe to help during the insertion itself so here we describe how to do that.

With the **ultrasound** it's vital to **orientate the probe correctly** and usually this will mean having the blue dot on the screen corresponding to the medial aspect of the picture. Ensure the depth of the picture is set so that you maximise the vessel size but can also see important local

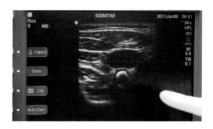

The finger is pointing to a circular structure with a white outline, this is the carotid artery which you will see is pulsating, the black blob above this is the jugular vein which is compressible with the probe

structures – namely the internal carotid artery and sternocleidomastoid. The vein is usually larger, lying more superficially and is compressible. The usual level of approach is at **C6**, at the **level of the cricoid** which you should be able to palpate and this corresponds to the angle between the sternal and clavicular heads of sternocleidomastoid. The internal jugular vein lies at this angle and runs inferolaterally to join the subclavian vein. The vein is found in the carotid sheath which contains the **internal carotid artery medially** and the **vagus nerve posteriorly**.

Keep the **probe perpendicular** to the skin, keeping the vessel in the middle of the screen, and infiltrate the local anaesthetic if indicated. Next, with the needle/cannula attached to the 5 ml syringe **puncture the skin** about 1 cm behind but in line with the middle of the probe. The angle of puncture is of debate but one way is to enter the skin at an angle of **45°** and for the puncture site to be a centimetre or two behind the probe. If the picture on the ultrasound shows the vein to be 1.5cm below the skin surface, then if you puncture the skin at a distance of 1.5cm above the probe at a 45° angle, it is much easier to enter the vessel.

Another tip when using ultrasound is to obtain a view that doesn't position the carotid artery directly below the internal jugular vein, thus minimising the risk of accidental arterial puncture. This may actually mean slowly rotating the probe medially until you have a clear view of vein superficially.

Advance the needle until you can **aspirate venous blood** freely and then, whilst holding the needle still, **remove the syringe** and **feed the guide wire, which should pass easily through the needle.** If the cannula method is used then the cannula is advanced into the vein and the needle withdrawn so the wire is fed into the cannula. The J-tip end is blunted and rounded to avoid damage to the vein but must be prepared by withdrawing the J into the plastic introducer – best done during your trolley set-up. This will minimise any blood flowing back from the needle as another bonus. The **wire should move freely** through the needle

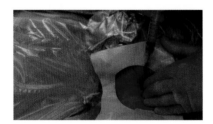

The needle and syringe are advanced until flashback of dark venous blood is aspirated

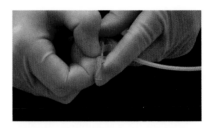

The guidewire has a J-tip, in order to aid insertion, it should be withdrawn first into the plastic holding device which straightens it out

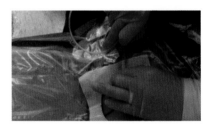

The guidewire being threaded through the needle

and no resistance should be encountered. **Don't force the wire through any resistance**. It may be that an assistant may need to provide downward traction on the ipsilateral arm to aid passage of the wire. Whilst passing the wire it's important to **keep an eye on the ECG** for ectopics or other rhythm disturbance caused by advancing the wire too far. Simply withdraw the wire a little should this be the case. The wire usually is marked at 10cm intervals with a line for each interval, e.g. 2 lines for 20cm. Once the wire is through, the **needle can be removed** while keeping the guidewire in the vessel. **Never let go of the guidewire**. The ultrasound can also be useful to see the wire in the vein and an in-plane view can be used to confirm the position of the wire more easily.

The next step is to **dilate the track** currently occupied by the wire. To allow passage of the dilator it's better to make a **small incision** in the skin with the supplied scalpel. Keep the blade facing outwards and make a small stab with intent with the non cutting edge of the blade sliding against the wire. You don't need to go deep, just enough to get through the skin – the dilator will dilate everything except tough skin. Now, **feed the dilator over the wire** and push the dilator through the skin. It isn't usually necessary to advance the dilator all the way- by using the ultrasound you already have an idea of the location of the vein and how

deep it lies. This is the point where gentle pressure is often needed to get the dilator through the skin and then into the vessel.

Now you are going to **exchange the dilator for the catheter**- have some sterile gauze to hand at the insertion site whilst removing the dilator and holding the wire steady. The **wire must be held in position** and not allowed to advance as the central line is threaded onto the wire, and as the **line is advanced through the skin**, ensure you still have the wire in one hand as the catheter is positioned. Depending on the habitus of the patient and the level of insertion, some of the catheter may be left outside the patient or it may be advanced to the hilt. **Remove the**

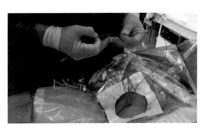

The dilator is removed and the catheter is threaded over the guidewire

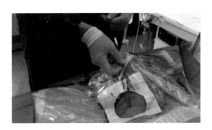

Make a small nick in the skin

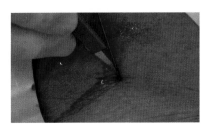

Thread the dilator over the guidewire

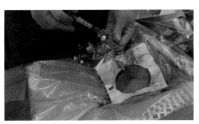

A syringe is attached to the port and the lumen can be aspirated and flushed

wire once the catheter is in position. Blood should flow back into the port where the wire once was. **Aspirate and flush each port with saline**, ensuring that each lumen is locked off to avoid air embolism.

Finally **secure the line** with either sutures, or as is more commonplace nowadays, custom-made fixation devices with skin preparation to allow the devices to stick properly. Another **transparent bio-occlusive dressing** is applied over the insertion site. A **chest x-ray** to confirm the position of the line should be performed as soon as possible and **transducing the line** to obtain a central venous waveform are the **gold standards** for confirming

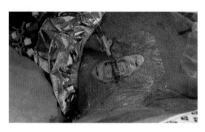

The drain secured in place

correct placement of the central line. A blood gas sample may also be of use.

Clean off all the skin prep and remove and discard your drapes. **Dispose of your sharps** (including the guidewire) immediately into a sharps bin. **Document the procedure** clearly in the notes.

OSCE checklist

- Positions patient correctly and exposes neck
- Understands role of duplex scanning
- Scrubs and dons appropriate sterile personal protective attire
- Assembles equipment correctly
- Cleans skin
- Creates sterile field
- Identifies carotid artery as landmark by palpation
- Inserts needle introducer
- Aspirates whilst advancing
- Aspirates venous blood
- Removes syringe whilst keeping needle still
- Threads guidewire through needle
- Removes the needle while keeping the guidewire still
- Makes a small nick in the skin

- Threads the dilator over the guidewire
- Removes the dilator
- Threads the central venous catheter over the guidewire
- Always keeps hold of the guidewire
- Removes the guidewire
- Aspirates blood from the lumen to confirm in vein
- Applies a 3-way port or hub to end of lumen
- Aspirates air from tap and flushes saline
- Attaches cap to port
- Secures catheter
- Applies occlusive dressing
- Washes hands
- Thanks patient
- Disposes of sharps and waste
- Documents procedure
- Provides postprocedure advice

14   Electrocardiogram

Video Time | 2 mins 58 s

Overview

Let's imagine you are the surgical F1, and one of your patients has recently returned from theatre following a lengthy femoropopliteal bypass. She complains of some mild chest discomfort and you, being the extraordinarily brilliant doctor that you are, remember well that vascular patients are especially prone to myocardial infarctions. The nurse is on her break. The other nurse is busy with a patient. Embarrassingly, you haven't performed an electrocardiogram (ECG) since third year, when once one of your hungover colleagues complained of palpitations during a clinical skills session. Not to worry. After watching this video, your ECG gremlins will be entirely exiled, and you will be as efficient as any cardiac technician.

Chest pain is by far the most frequent indication for performing an ECG, it's extremely useful and provides an almost instantaneous electrical trace to identify ischaemia related changes. But remember that other cardiac or respiratory symptoms such as palpitations, tachycardia, sudden shortness of breath and non-specific 'unwellness' (especially where no other cause can be identified) can help you identify silent myocardial infarctions.

Electrical changes within the myocardium can be detected and visualised using an ECG. Electrodes placed around the heart allow you to 'look' at electrical activity from different angles. Interpretation of these patterns can give clues or even diagnose underlying pathology.

The misuse of the word 'lead' can cause confusion. Often it's used synonymously to describe the actual wires that connect the patient to the ECG machine. In reality, you should realise that the ECG consists of 10 electrodes and wires

How to Perform Clinical Procedures, First Edition. Matthew Stephenson, Joshua Shur and John Black.

which generate 12 views of the heart or 'leads'. This is explained below and demonstrated in the accompanying video.

Each electrode is positioned to create 'leads' looking at the heart from a multitude of directions. ECG interpretation is easy if you remember the directions from which the various 'leads' look at the heart. Six standard 'leads' are obtained from the 4 limb electrodes, and can be thought of as looking at the heart in vertical planes from the sides and the patient's feet. Broadly speaking, leads I and aVL look at the lateral left ventricle, leads II, III and aVF at the inferior surface, and lead aVR looks at the right atrium.

The 6 numbered V leads (V1–V6) look at the heart in a horizontal plane, from the front and the lateral left side. More specifically, leads V1 and V2 look at the right ventricle, leads V3 and V4 look at the myocardial septum between the ventricles and anterior wall of the left ventricle, and finally, leads V5 and V6 look at the anterior and lateral walls of the left ventricle. As with the limb leads, due to positioning, all leads show a variation on the ECG pattern. However, each lead pattern is of a similar characteristic in different individuals deemed to have a normal heart.

The grid below represents the common indications warranting an ECG.

Indications	Contraindications	Complications
• Chest pain • Palpitations • Dyspnoea • Hypotension • Hypertension • Electrolyte disturbance • Presyncopal episode • Syncope • Trauma • Preoperative (routine) • Postoperative (routine) • 'Sick' patients • Diabetic patients	• None (although it may be difficult to obtain an accurate trace in the tremulous/ confused/agitated patient)	• None

Procedure

Make sure you have the **correct patient**, for the **correct procedure**. Check for any **allergies** (unlikely to be an issue in this procedure), and that you have confirmed the **indication;** excluded any **contraindications; explained** the procedure and taken **consent**. Now **wash your hands**!

Assemble all of your equipment on a trolley away from the patient and this usually all comes together on an ECG trolley. You will need everything in the equipment textbox. The ECG recorder may vary from trust to trust dependent on the manufacturer, but the principles remain the same with all machines. **Check that the ECG machine works**, and that the trace **printer is loaded** with the correct paper.

The **chest should be exposed**. For men, this is relatively straightforward – it usually involves them taking off their shirt. For a female undergoing an ECG this may involve requesting them to remove their bra should their breasts prove to be obstructive. Breast magnitude and laxity is highly variable amongst the population, and you should do your best to accommodate the varying anatomy. Appreciate that at times, particularly in the elderly population, the Cooper's ligaments are just not as efficient as they used to be! Therefore, in such instances it may require your chaperone (of paramount importance if you are a chap) to elevate the mammary glands in order to oppose gravity and ensure correct placement.

Position the patient to 45° and encourage them to **relax** to prevent interference from muscle tremor. Obviously, in some circumstances, the patient may have an involuntary tremor. Whilst this can be problematic, you strive to make the best of a bad situation – and consider it later when interpreting the ECG.

In the event of your patient's chest having an appearance of the forest of dean, you must counsel them on the need for **hair removal**. This can be effectively achieved either by manually shaving the patient if necessary. Hair can cause poor coupling between skin and electrode, thus giving a noisy trace.

You're now ready to **attach the electrode stickers** to the patient. This involves an appreciation of bony landmarks and basic surface anatomy. You will require 10 adhesive electrodes in total. These are standardised self-adhesive pads, with coupling media embedded into them. They include a small flap which the wire clips to. **Start with the limbs**, before finally placing the **chest electrodes** (which require a little more precision and skill).

With the **skin file** on the index finger of your dominant hand, remove any excess shaved hair and exfoliate surface skin cells (in the emergency setting this is rarely done), before placing an adhesive electrode over the **bony prominence of** the **right humeral head**. Place a second electrode over the **prominence of the left humeral head**, using an identical skin prep technique. The third electrode is placed over the lateral aspect, just proximal to the **lateral malleolus of the left leg**, and a fourth is placed in a similar position over on the **right leg**. Try to avoid thick muscle. Some place electrodes 3 and 4 over the left and right lower abdomen instead of the legs.

With your skin file still on your index finger, you are ready to palpate, prepare the skin and place the chest electrodes. Identify the **angle of Louis** at the sternum, and find the second rib to the right of the sternum. Count down and place the **V1** electrode in the **right 4th intercostal space** (in between ribs 4 and 5), just to the right of the sternum. Staying in the same axial plane, place the **V2** electrode in the **left 4th intercostal space**, just to the left of the sternum.

Skip to V4, and place this one space lower in the **5th intercostal space** (in between ribs 5 and 6), in the **mid clavicular line**. This allows you to place **V3 equidistant between V2 and V4**. Place **V5** horizontally with V4, again heading laterally, in the left **anterior axilliary line**. Finally place **V6** horizontally at the same axial level with V4 and V5 in the **mid axillary line**.

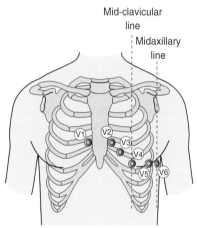

Diagram of ECG lead placement positions

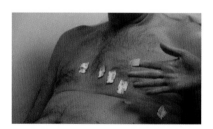

On the technician's finger tip is mounted a skin file to exfoliate the skin before pad placement; this is often not performed in practice on the wards and in emergencies but does help skin contact

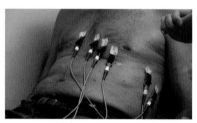

All the chest leads connected

Once you have placed your electrodes in the correct anatomical positions, you're ready to **attach the wires** which relay the electrical information to the recorder. It's worth ensuring that the electrodes are in the correct place before attaching the wires.

Similarly starting with the limb wires, **first** wire is usually labeled '**RA**' and is **red** in appearance. This clips onto the electrode placed on the **right arm**. Next, attach the **second** wire or '**LA**' to the **left arm** electrode. This is **yellow**. The **third** wire, '**LL**' is **green** and clips onto the electrode of the **left lower leg**. The **fourth** limb wire is **black** and labeled '**RL**'. This is attached to the remaining limb electrode of the **right leg**. Well done. The limb electrodes and wires are done.

Move swiftly on to the **chest wires**: The wire labelled **V1** attaches to the **V1 electrode**, wire V2 to the V2 electrode and so forth and so on, until you have attached the 6th and final chest lead (**V1: Red, V2: Yellow, V3: Green, V4: Brown, V5: Black, V6 Violet**). Note that the colours of all the wires are standard across Europe (the USA have a different colour coding system). You are now ready to proceed to obtaining your reading.

Ensure the recorder is turned to the 'on setting'. **Calibrate** your machine using the digital display if necessary although most modern machines tend to calibrate automatically. Most ECG machines now have an electronic representation of your 12 leads. The internationally accepted calibration is set to a standard: A signal of 1 millivolt should move the stylus vertically 1 cm (or 2 large squares). This calibration signal usually appears at the beginning of the trace with every record. The paper speed should also be set to 25 mm per second.

Ensure the patient is **lying as still as possible** and once you have a clear digital representation of your 12 leads, the machine will either automatically capture a trace or you simply **press the button** that states 'Start' or 'Capture' or something similar – it will be obvious, and even if there are other buttons on the machine, you're unlikely to need to use them. You just need the Start button. If the patient is moving a lot, it may refuse to do this as the machine may be equipped with an interference sensor, or you may just get a very useless printout. Some machines have a helpful sensor that tells you when the best possible trace has been obtained.

Remember to **label the ECG** with time and date and the patient's details and you should also note down whether they were having any symptoms at the time of the ECG, for example 'chest pain'. Needless to say really, but you've then got to interpret the ECG and act on it!

To complete the procedure, **unclip the wires** and **remove the electrodes**, offering the patient a tissue to wipe away any conductance gel residue. **Wash your hands**, **thank** the patient and **document** the procedure in the patient's notes.

Stepwise approach of ECG analysis: suggested

The normal ECG:	P wave	Width: <2.5 mm
		Height << 0.11 seconds in lead II
	P–R interval	0.12–02 sec. (3–5 small squares)
	QRS complex	Width: <0.12 sec. (<3 small squares)
	ST segment	Isoelectric–in line with successive heart beats.
	T wave	Upright except in aVR, III and V1 50% of the QRS.
	AT interval	QTC = QT/R–R interval Men: <450 mS Women: <470 MS

Cardiac axis:	Rate	300/R–R interval. Normal = 60–100 bpm
	Rhythm	Sinus rhythm if: 1. P waves precedes very QRS 2. Regluar R–R interval
	Axis	1. Find the most isoelectric limb lead 2. The cardiac axis lies 90 degrees to this in the positive direction.
	P waves	Broad or Bifid = P mitrale Peaked = P pulmonale
	QRS complex	Broad = LBBB RSR in V1 with slurred S in V6 = RBBB.
	ST segment	Elevation >1 mm in two contiguous limb leads or >2 mm in 2 chest leads + myocardial infarction-for PCI and thrombolysis.
	T wave	Can be inverted in aVR V1 and III
	QT interval QTc = QT/RR	A borderline normal Women: 431–450 mS Men: 451–470 mS

	II	III
Normal axis	+	+
LAD	+	−
RAD	−	+/

A stepwise approach for junior doctors (Guy's and St Thomas' Hospitals; NHS Foundation trust)

Atrial flutter

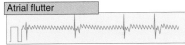

- A characteristic "sawtooth" or "picket-fence" waveform
- Usually about 300 bpm
- Flutter is often accompanied with 2:1 block and so you may find a ventricular rate of 150bpm

Atrial fibrillation

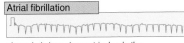

- Irregularly irregular ventricular rhythm
- Fast AF > 100 bpm

LBBB

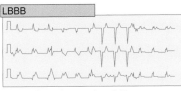

- The QRS duration must be ≥0.12s
- There should be a QS or rS complex in lead V1
- There should be a monophasic R wave in leads I and V6 (W in V1 and M in V6)

Complete heart block

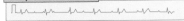

- The P waves with a regular P to P interval represents the first rhythm
- The QRS complexes with regular R to R interval represent the second rhythm
- The PR interval will be variable, as the hallmark of complete heart block is no apparent relationship between P waves and QRS complexes

Acute anterior MI

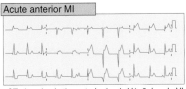

- ST elevation in the anterior leads V1–6, I and aVL
- Reciprocal ST depression in the inferior leads

Ventricular tachycardia

- A wide QRS is ventricular tachycardia till proven otherwise
- P waves are hidden in the QRS

Common ECG examples

OSCE checklist

- Positions patient correctly with chest exposed
- Attaches limb lead stickers correctly
- Uses skin prep correctly
- Uses bony landmarks to identify chest lead positions
- Attaches chest lead stickers correctly
- Connects leads correctly
- Checks calibration
- Obtains trace adequately
- Washes hands
- Thanks patient
- Documents procedure
- Provides postprocedure advice

15 Endotracheal Intubation

Reshma Woograsingh and Christopher Parnell

Video Time | 3 mins 53 s

Overview

Endotracheal intubation is a core skill for anaesthetic trainees and intensive care doctors. Some A&E doctors may also perform this procedure in the acute setting and indeed some paramedics may arrive in the resuscitation bay having intubated a patient in cardiac arrest. Many patients on intensive care are also intubated and as a junior working in this environment it's important to know the basics as to how an endotracheal tube is placed and how to assess correct insertion.

By definition, endotracheal intubation describes a definitive airway whereby there is minimal risk of aspiration of gastric contents, which may be the case if a laryngeal mask airway is used for example. Sometimes it's not always possible to intubate a patient due to abnormalities in the anatomy of the airway, which may be due to body habitus or pathology of a patient, and this is known as a 'can't intubate' scenario.

Depending on whether you are able to ventilate the patient, the next step is to use an alternative airway (such as a laryngeal mask airway) or adjuncts (includinga Guedel/oropharyngeal airway) and consider allowing the patient to wake up. If you are unable to ventilate the patient, this is obviously a more serious situation, and early consideration to emergency airway interventions such as a needle cricothyroidotomy should be given. These are described by the Difficult Airway Society guidelines for airway management.

How to Perform Clinical Procedures, First Edition. Matthew Stephenson, Joshua Shur and John Black.
© 2013 John Wiley & Sons, Ltd. Published 2013 by John Wiley & Sons, Ltd.

Indications	Contraindications	Complications
• Rapid sequence induction – an anaesthetic technique for securing an airway quickly in emergency situations • Cardiac arrest (although not shown to alter outcome) • Patients undergoing intra-abdominal and cardiothoracic surgery • Patients with significant reflux undergoing general anaesthetic • Instances where significant movement during surgery or lateral/prone positions may disrupt a less adequately secured airway.	• No specific contraindications but take care if previously documented difficult intubation or airway abnormalities	• Oesophageal intubation • Endobronchial intubation • 'Can't intubate' or 'can't intubate, can't ventilate' scenario

Procedure

Make sure you have the **correct patient**, for the **correct procedure**. Check for any **allergies**, and that you have confirmed the **indication;** excluded any **contraindications; explained** the procedure and taken **consent**. Now **wash your hands**!

Assemble all of your equipment on a sterile trolley away from the patient. You will need everything in the equipment textbox.

Prepare your equipment. The endotracheal tube is sized according to the internal diameter – a size 8 is denoted as a #8.0 – and corresponds to the internal diameter of the tube. A size 8.0 is usually used for males and a 7.0 for females. It is curved concave upwards and has a cuff attached to a pilot tube to which a syringe

Equipment you need (on a sterile tray/trolley)

- Laryngoscope handle
- Laryngoscope blade – MacIntosh
- Gum elastic bougie
- Guedel (oropharyngeal) airway
- Endotracheal tubes in a variety of sizes
- 10 ml syringe
- Cuff pressure monitor
- Facemask
- Suction
- Difficult airway equipment on standby
  - McCoy blade
  - Video laryngoscope, e.g. MacGrath
  - Laryngeal mask airway

can be attached and inflated with air. **Ensure the endotracheal tube cuff is patent**, inflates adequately and is coated

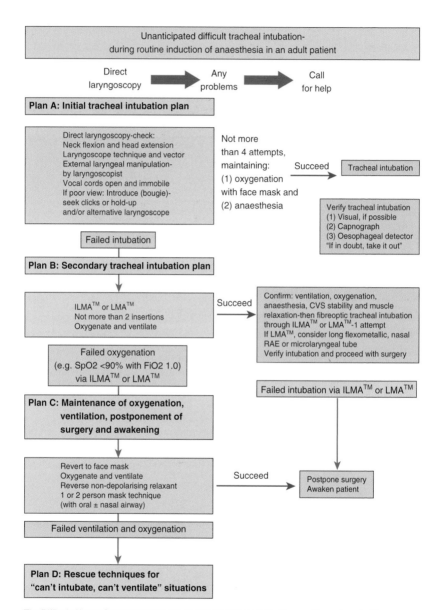

The Difficult Airway Society guidelines for airway management. (*Source:* Reproduced with permission of Difficult Airway Society)

with a water-based lubricant. **Check your laryngoscope** blade light source is working by attaching to the handle and testing the fibreoptic light source.

In the video we show how to intubate a patient undergoing elective surgery and demonstrate a straightforward induction of anaesthesia in order to provide conditions for intubation. The **patient is attached to monitoring** in accordance with the AAGBI (Association of Anaesthetists of Great Britain and Ireland) guidelines – specifically ECG, SpO2 and

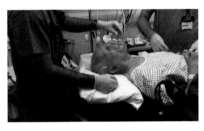

The patient is supine with the head appropriately positioned.The patient is being preoxgenated

BP measurement. **Intravenous access is secured** before proceeding.

It's important to **preoxygenate** patients – this allows denitrogenation of the functional residual capacity of the lungs and will buy time in the event of a difficult intubation.

Next, **the patient is anaesthetised**-this usually involves administration of fentanyl (a potent opioid) and then an induction agent – usually propofol, titrated to effect. The result of this is anaesthesia with resultant loss of consciousness and apnoea. The position of the patient is paramount to success. The patient should be positioned in what is classically described as a 'sniffing the morning air' position. This essentially means that the head is slightly flexed while the neck is extended.

It's prudent to **check you can ventilate the patient** before administering a **muscle relaxant** which will paralyse the patient and allow passage of the tube through the vocal cords. The patient is

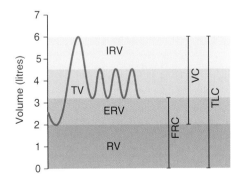

Spirometry showing

TV-tidal volume
IRV-inspiratory reserve volume
ERV-expiratory reserve volume
RV-residual volume
FRC-functional residual capacity
VC-vital capacity
TLC-total lung capacity

kept asleep using volatile agents delivered through the anaesthetic machine as long as ventilation is maintained.

Muscle relaxants vary in time to onset for intubating conditions but usually take between 60 and 90 seconds to achieve their effect. Then a **laryngoscope**, which is a left-handed instrument (regardless of one's handedness!), **is inserted into the mouth with the tip in the vallecula**; if a MacIntosh blade is used, the tongue is swept to the left of the oral cavity. In the video a MacGrath video-laryngoscope is used; other videolaryngoscopes are available where there is no need for the tongue to be displaced in this manner.

Next you need to **view the vocal cords** – this is done by displacing the laryngoscope anteriorly. It's important not to damage teeth or soft tissues around the oral cavity, so your left wrist should be kept in line with your forearm and the direction of displacement is in line with your hand and forearm and the laryngoscope handle. You should see the vocal cords and **the view is graded using the Cormack and Lehane classification** as follows. Suction of secretions may help your view!

The **endotracheal tube is passed between the vocal cords** and the black marker on the tube indicates where the tube should lie level with the vocal cords. Depending on the laryngoscopic view **a Bougie may be useful**. This is a smaller stylet which is slightly curved anteriorly to slip under the egiglottis and into the trachea. If a bougie is used, successful passage into the trachea will be felt as tracheal 'clicks' as the bougie passes

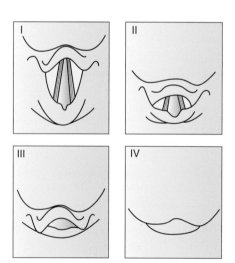

Grade I: The vocal cords are seen fully with the epiglottis superiorly-i.e. the glottis is seen
Grade II: The glottis partially seen- the anterior vocal fold is obscured
Grade III: Only the epiglottis is seen with corniculate cartilage
Grade IV: Neither the glottis or corniculate cartilage is seen

Classification of laryngoscopy views

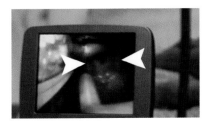

The view of the cords with the laryngoscope. This would be a Grade II intubation. The yellow structure is the bougie

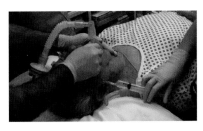

The syringe is used to inflate the cuff

over the tracheal rings. The laryngoscope remains inserted as the endotracheal tube is passed over the bougie and held in place whilst correct positioning of the tube is confirmed. You may need to twist the tube 90° to aid passage into the trachea if using a bougie. Once the tube is in place, remove the laryngoscope and bougie and **inflate the cuff** with air. The cuff pressure can be specifically measured with a pressure gauge and adjusted accordingly.

Attach the breathing circuit and **assess correct positioning** by ventilating – specifically: chest rise and fall, capnography (which detects CO_2 expired by the patient) and auscultate lung fields for equal air entry. If the tube is passed too far, then it's likely that the tube will pass endobronchially into the right main bronchus due to the anatomy of the bronchial tree.

Secure the tube position with a tie or tape. Ensure that waste is disposed of, wash your hands and the procedure is documented, usually on an anaesthetic chart.

OSCE checklist

- Assembles equipment correctly
- Checks laryngoscope
- Preoxygenates patient
- Lowers bed
- Administers analgesia
- Administers general anaesthetic
- Checks level of anaesthesia
- Performs head tilt and chin lift
- Inserts oropharyngeal airway
- Checks ability to ventilate patient
- Uses laryngoscope correctly
- Visualises epiglottis
- Visualises vocal cords
- Uses bougie to aid intubation (optional)
- Intubates trachea successfully
- Inflates cuff
- Confirms correct position
- Ties ET tube in place
- Washes hands
- Disposes of waste
- Documents procedure in notes

16 Epidural

Reshma Woograsingh and Christopher Parnell

Video Time | 6 mins 59 s

Overview

Epidurals are commonly used to provide analgesia on the labour ward for parturients and also in theatres as an adjunct to general anaesthesia. They are useful for analgesia postoperatively for a wide variety of surgical procedures, for example, laparotomies, lower limb surgery for hips and knees or vascular grafts. So, as a surgical junior doctor, you are very likely to happen upon a patient who has one! Whilst it is usually the Pain Team or anaesthetists who will help manage epidurals on the ward, it's worth knowing a bit about them as you are likely to be the first port of call.

The advantage of using an epidural to help with pain relief means that a patient often requires less opiate medication, so reducing the side-effects of nausea/vomiting, constipation or pruritis. In patients who have undergone thoraco-abdominal surgery with a large incision, an effective epidural results in less impact on their respiratory system: if they are comfortable then they will be able to take deep breaths and cough, thus reducing the risk of atelectasis and a chest infection brewing. They are more likely to mobilise effectively and keep the physiotherapists happy too!

One of the most common side-effects of epidurals is hypotension. This is due to the local anaesthetic that is infused through the epidural catheter, which causes sympathetic blockade as well as analgesia. This can often be treated by simply administering a fluid challenge and giving consideration to reducing the rate of infusion of local anaesthetic only once the block has been assessed. The most common infusion of local anaesthetic used is bupivicaine 0.1% combined with fentanyl 2 mcg/ml, although this can vary between hospitals. Even though fentanyl is an opiate, the incidence of side-effects from this method of administration is less than if opiates were given intravenously or orally.

How to Perform Clinical Procedures, First Edition. Matthew Stephenson, Joshua Shur and John Black.
© 2013 John Wiley & Sons, Ltd. Published 2013 by John Wiley & Sons, Ltd.

Indications	Contraindications	Complications
• Perioperative analgesia • Peripartum analgesia • Perioperative anaesthesia, e.g. Caesarian section	• Coagulopathy • Localised skin infection over insertion site • Raised intracranial pressure • Hypovolaemia • Fixed cardiac output states, e.g. aortic stenosis, HOCM (relative) • Preexisting neurological deficit (relative) – be sure to document before you do the procedure!	• Dural (tap and postdural puncture headache PDPH) • Venous puncture • Neuropraxia • Epidural haematoma • Epidural abscess • Meningitis, arachnoiditis • Medication side effects: Hypotension Nausea/vomiting Pruritis

Procedure

Make sure you have the **correct patient**, for the **correct procedure**. Check for any **allergies**, and that you have confirmed the **indication;** excluded any **contraindications; explained** the procedure and taken **consent**. Now **wash your hands**!

Assemble all of your equipment on a sterile trolley away from the patient. You will need everything in the equipment textbox.

The procedure is performed usually in an awake patient who is sitting upright, although sometimes in theatre a patient may be anaesthetised first and placed in a lateral position to insert the epidural. It's useful to know if you're brushing too close to nerves, which can only really be done in an awake patient! A 'loss-of-resistance' technique is employed to identify the epidural/extradural space and a catheter is threaded into this space to administer the local anaesthetic. A little anatomy revision before we start, then!.

Equipment you need (on a sterile tray/trolley)

- Cleaning solution
- Tuohey needle (usually 16G)
- Epidural catheter
- Hub to attach catheter
- Filter to attach to hub (0.2 micron) with cap
- Loss-of-resistance syringe
- Introducer
- Local anaesthetic, e.g. 1% lidocaine
- 25G needle for initial LA infiltration
- 21G needle for further infiltration
- 5 ml syringe
- Normal saline for flush
- Sterile gauze
- Sterile dressing / fixation device

The epidural space lies outside the dural sac which contains cerebrospinal fluid (CSF) and spinal cord or cauda equina, depending on the level of insertion. It contains loosely bound fat and an extensive venous plexus as well as the nerve roots. As an epidural is inserted

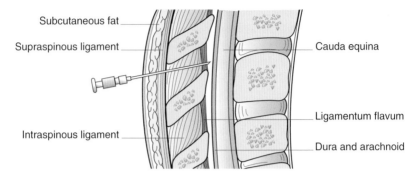

Subcutaneous fat

Supraspinous ligament

Cauda equina

Ligamentum flavum

Intraspinous ligament

Dura and arachnoid

The layers that the epidural needle must pass to reach the epidural space

there are several layers to pass through: skin, subcutaneous fat, supraspinous ligament, interspinous ligament and ligamentum flavum. It's a space under negative pressure, which is why a loss-of-resistance technique is used to identify it.

So now for the actual procedure! Having prepared your kit, **ensure the patient is positioned appropriately**. This will mean having them sat on the edge of the bed with their feet on a fixed surface, for example a stool or chair. If you ask them to have the back of their knees at the edge of the bed and their feet flat on the stool then this will improve stability. Often, a pillow is used for them to wrap their arms around and then they should curve their back out like an angry cat, or a banana. Ideally they should have their chin on their chest and shoulders relaxed and the most important aspect is that their vertebral spines are as close to the midline as possible. The whole point of this is to facilitate easy insertion and open up the intervertebral spaces as much as possible.

Next, **palpate the spaces to find the level** that you want to insert the epidural. For labour ward patients L2/3 or L3/4 is ideal. Higher levels of insertion are needed for more extensive operations, for example a laparotomy incision would often require an epidural at T9/10. An imaginary line joining the tops of the iliac crests corresponds to the body of the L4 vertebra, so count up from there. You may wish to mark the spot by indenting the skin with the blunt end of a needle or simply mark it.

Now **get scrubbed and prepare your equipment**. You should draw up

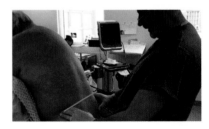

Positioning of the patient and identification of the bony landmarks

your local anaesthetic and have the smaller 21G needle attached to it. Then your epidural catheter should be attached to the hub and filter and flushed with saline to ensure patency of these. Prepare the epidural needle and attach the wings.

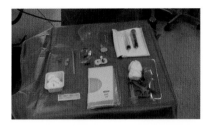

The equipment trolley set up

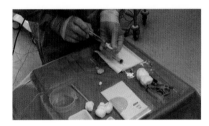

The catheter hub has been attached to the catheter and the syringe is then attached in order to flush it

Clean the skin with an appropriate agent, (current best practice is to use 0.5% chlorhexidine, as more concentrated solutions can cause arachnoiditis) and then **apply the sterile drape** – the aperture drapes are ideal and often come in the pack. Next, find your mark, and **infiltrate the local anaesthetic**, first with the narrower needle to make a skin bleb, then deeper using the longer and

wider 18G needle. Be mindful of the body habitus of your patient as to the depth of needle insertion and don't forget to warn your patient of a sharp scratch – they can't see what you're doing!

Now **insert the epidural needle into the skin** in the midline and then into the ligaments. You may find that sometimes a paramedian approach is used. The epidural needle is known as a Tuohy needle and has a curved tip called a Huber tip.

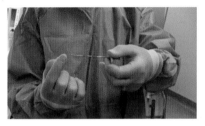

The Tuohy needle

This is blunted and should be pointing rostrally (towards the head) so as to aid passage of the epidural catheter. The angle of insertion will vary depending on the level of insertion, lumbar spaces being more horizontal as compared to thoracic ones. The needle will hold steady by itself in the skin in the interspinous ligament, usually 2–3 cm from the skin surface. Then, **remove the obturator from the epidural needle** and **attach the loss-of-resistance syringe** to the end of the epidural needle.

Now, if you apply pressure onto the end of the syringe you will find resistance from the ligament. **Advance the**

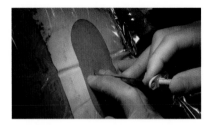

The epidural needle entering the skin

epidural needle by 1 mm and **check again for loss-of-resistance**. As the ligamentum flavum is reached, the resistance will increase further. Continue careful advancement, checking each time. You can always remove the syringe if you feel you may have advanced too far and breached the dural sac. This will be pretty obvious as you will get a gush of CSF onto the floor! In which case remove the Tuohy from the patient.

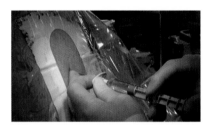

The loss-of-resistance syringe is attached to the epidural needle

Once loss-of-resistance is achieved as saline flows easily into the epidural space, carefully **remove the syringe** from the Tuohy needle and **attach the introducer** device before threading the epidural catheter. It should pass easily and not encoun-

ter resistance. The catheter is marked at 1 cm intervals with two lines at 10 cm, 3 at 15 cm and a larger mark at 20 cm. Given that the needle shaft is 8 cm and the hub is 2 cm, note how deep the epidural space is and **thread enough catheter** into the space. Then remove the needle, whilst maintaining the position of the catheter – you should push forward a little with the catheter as you remove the needle.

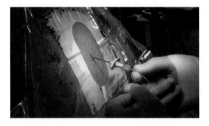

The epidural catheter is threaded though the needle

Now, you need to make sure that the right amount of catheter is left in the space. It is common practice to leave 4–5 cm in. So if the loss-of-resistance was at 4 cm depth, then the mark on the catheter at the skin should be 8 or 9 cm. Try 9 cm first and you can also check for a drop in the meniscus – this wasn't in the video but is one way of checking that the catheter is in

One other method you may encounter for advancing the epidural needle is to apply constant pressure to the syringe to advance the needle whilst maintaining stability of the needle with the other hand as a 'brake' to avoid rapid advancement once the epidural space is found.

the correct space. If you hold the free end of the flushed catheter above the level of insertion, the column of saline should fall. You can also check for inadvertent venous puncture by holding the free end below the level of insertion and observe if fluid comes out of the catheter. Definitively, **the hub should be attached and aspirated** with a syringe to **ensure no blood or cerebrospinal fluid** is found.

Attach the filter and the epidural cap. Next **dress the area** after cleaning any blood or remaining cleaning solution with sterile gauze. There are some custom-made fixation devices available but this will be guided by local policy. Ideally you should still be able to see the area of insertion once the dressing is applied. Make one final check by injecting saline with minimal pressure into the space. The other part of the catheter is fixed to the back in an upwards direction so as to leave the filter and hub over the patients shoulder for ease of access.

Finally **clear away your sharps** and equipment and **document the procedure** clearly in the notes.

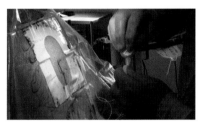

The antibacterial filter is being screwed on to the hub

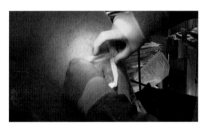

A simple transparent adhesive dressing

OSCE Checklist

- Positions patient correctly
- Identifies bony landmarks correctly
- Confirms in midline
- Marks chosen site
- Scrubs and dons appropriate sterile personal protective attire
- Assembles equipment correctly
- Checks expiry dates of injectables
- Flushes catheter with normal saline
- Cleans skin
- Applies sterile drape with aperture
- Warns about a 'sharp scratch'
- Infiltrates with local anaesthetic
- Injects local anaesthetic – deep
- Inserts the epidural (Tuohy) needle
- Applies gentle pressure and confirms resistance
- Removes obturator
- Applies gentle pressure on syringe and confirms resistance
- Gently advances needle whilst applying pressure on syringe
- Identifies reduced resistance

17 Flexible Nasendoscopy

Bertram Fu and Meredydd Harries

Video Time | 3 mins 16 s

Overview

Performing Flexible Nasendoscopy (FNE) is an integral part of completing an Ear, Nose and Throat (ENT) examination. Although at first glance it may look daunting to junior doctors and patients, it's actually a relatively straightforward skill that most can acquire given the correct instructions and opportunity to practise. In contrast to most endoscopic examinations in medicine (i.e. bronchoscopy, gastroscopy, colonscopy, and cystoscopy) where sedation or general anaesthesia is commonly required, FNE is often done in the clinic or ward settings with no sedation and usually no local anaesthesia.

In skilled hands, the procedure should take no longer than 1-2 minutes and is therefore well tolerated by the majority of our patients.

FNE allows one to have an unprecedented view of the upper aerodigestive tract and is therefore helpful in the diagnosis and management of a wide variety of ENT conditions.

There are many indications for 'scoping' an ENT patient, both in the elective and emergency settings. The following table, (The structures and pathology examined during flexible nasendoscopy), summarises some of the common scenarios where FNE may be useful.

Procedure

Make sure you have the **correct patient**, for the **correct procedure**. Check for any **allergies**, and that you have confirmed the **indication;** excluded any **contraindications; explained** the procedure and taken **consent**. Now **wash your hands**!

Assemble all of your equipment on a trolley away from the patient. Be sure to give clear instructions throughout the procedure.

How to Perform Clinical Procedures, First Edition. Matthew Stephenson, Joshua Shur and John Black.
© 2013 John Wiley & Sons, Ltd. Published 2013 by John Wiley & Sons, Ltd.

The structures and pathology examined during flexible nasendoscopy

Sites	Presentations	Structures to be assessed
Ears	Hearing loss from unilateral glue ear in an adult	Postnasal space and eustachian tube orifices
	Eustachian tube dysfunction	Postnasal space and eustachian tube orifices
Nose and nasopharynx	Epistaxis	Nasal cavities, septum, turbinates, meati and postnasal space
	Rhinosinusitis, allergic rhinitis, nasal polyposis	Nasal cavities, septum, turbinates, meati, postnasal space and nasal polyps
	Choanal atresia	Posterior choanae
	Septal perforation	Septum
Oral cavity and oropharynx	Impacted fish bone	Tongue base, vallecula, tonsils, hypopharynx
	Quinsy	Supraglottis
	Snoring (during induced sleep in general anaesthesia)	Soft palate, uvula, tongue base collapse
Larynx	Dysphonia (hoarseness)	Supraglottis, glottis and subglottis
	Dysphagia (swallowing difficulty)	Supraglottis, glottis, subglottis, and piriform fossae
	Stridor (noisy breathing)	Epiglottis, supraglottis, glottis, and subglottis
	Laryngopharyngeal reflux	Glottis
Head and neck	Pre or post thyroidectomy patients	Vocal cords

Equipment you need

- Light source – portable with battery supply or 'light box' with AC mains supply
- Flexible nasendoscope
- Decontamination wipe-system or sheaths
- Gloves
- Optional: aqueous gel Co-Phenylcaine

Connect the nasendoscope (the 'scope') to the light source. Put on the sheath for decontamination purposes if required. Otherwise, check and **adjust the focus** of the scope until a clear view is obtained.

Tilt the nasal tip of the patient's nose up and have a look at the anterior nasal cavities. Assess and **decide which nostril** will give you the easiest access for the passage of the scope. Inserting the scope on the side with a dislocated columella, deviated anterior nasal septum, and/or hypertrophied inferior turbinate will often make the procedure more difficult and unpleasant for the patient.

Spray the Co-Phenylcaine (a mixture solution of Lidocaine and Phenylephrine) directly inside the nasal cavity or soak it on a small piece of cotton ball before leaving it inside the nose for 5 minutes if necessary.

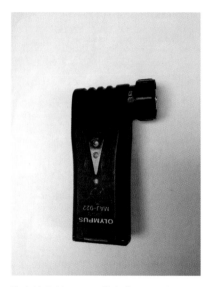

Portable light source with battery supply

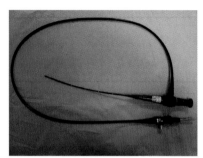

A flexible nasendoscope

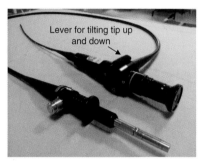

Lever for tilting tip up and down

A close-up view showing the lever controlling the position of the tip of the scope

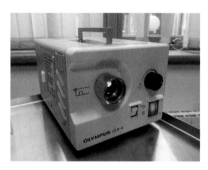

'Light Box' with AC mains supply

This may be a good idea especially when you are doing FNE on a child, a less tolerant adult patient, or in the presence of anatomical obstruction where access is limited. One can use up to a maximum of 8 sprays in an adult or child over 12 years.

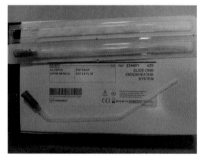

Disposable decontamination sheath

This is, however, not required in the majority of patients in experienced hands

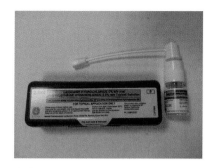

Co-Phenylcaine spray

anti-mist preparation will be required, which can be both difficult and expensive to obtain, hence the authors' preference for simple measures.

The tip of the scope can move in two directions by manipulating the lever with the index finger. Some prefer to hold the scope 'up-side-down' in which case the lever can be moved with the thumb. By combining this movement with rotation of the scope, one can in theory direct the scope in any angle.

as one can accurately direct the tip of the scope into clear spaces inside the nasal cavity without touching or traumatising the septum or inferior turbinate. In fact, a randomised controlled trial by Frosh AC *et al.* (1998)* has shown that the routine use of local anaesthesia is not only of no value, but actually makes the experience worse for the patient!

Ask the patient to **open his/her mouth** and **place the end of the scope below or on the tongue** for 5–10 seconds. This will warm the lens and allow the distal 2 cm of the scope to be covered with the patient's own saliva, which will act as both a lubricant and an excellent anti-mist to the lens. Others may wish to use aqueous gel as a lubricant. However, this can often smear across the lens and obscure the view. In addition, a separate

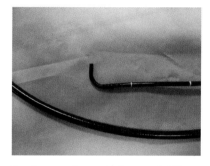

Tip of scope going maximally upwards 90°

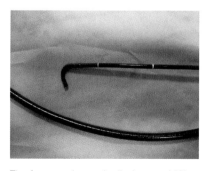

Tip of scope going maximally downward 90°

*Frosh AC, Jayaraj S, Porter G, Almeyda J (1998) Is local anaesthesia actually beneficial in flexible fibreoptic nasendoscopy? *Clin Otolaryngol Allied Sci* **23**(3): 259–62.

Ask the patient to breathe through his/her mouth and **insert the tip** of the scope horizontally into the nasal cavity. Try to stay low on the floor of the nasal cavity below the inferior turbinate or between the septum and the inferior turbinate while advancing the scope. Again, try to avoid touching the septum and the inferior turbinate with the tip of the scope as described above in order to minimise any pain or discomfort.

Look for the inferior turbinate, change the direction of the scope and **keep advancing the scope**. You can also examine the septum, middle turbinate and the middle meatus if indicated. At the posterior limit of the nasal cavity, the adenoid can be visualised in the postnasal space in children and the Eustachian tube orifices can be seen in both children and adults.

At this point, **turn the scope 90° downwards** and ask the patient to **breathe through his/her nose**. This will move the soft palate and uvula away and allow you to visualise the oropharynx from above. **Keep advancing** the scope for another 2–3 cm and ask the patient to **protrude his/her tongue out**. This will allow you to visualise the tongue base, vallecula and the supraglottis.

If the view is obscured while the tip of the scope is inside the oropharynx, ask the patient to swallow in order to 'wipe' the lens clean with the mucosal lining. Asking the patient to **take deep breaths in and out** (abduction) and say 'eeee' (adduction) will allow you to assess the position and movement of the vocal cords.

In addition, some practitioners may also ask the patient to **puff out his/her cheeks** and/or turning his/her head to one side and then the other side in order to examine the piriform fossae and the postcricoid areas. Some may even go on to advance the scope into the upper oesophagus while asking the patient to swallow. This will however trigger the gag reflex which is unpleasant in the majority of patients. This is therefore not practised routinely.

If the scope is connected to a camera and a stack system, you may wish to **take a video** of the examination in electronic file format or alternatively **freeze frame** a clinical photograph for documentation or educational purposes (i.e. in a posttreatment laryngeal cancer follow-up patient).

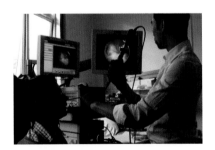

A patient is being scoped in the clinic. The scope is attached to the camera and stack system where electronic video and picture recordings can be obtained for clinical records

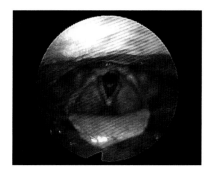

Endoscopic view of the larynx

Once you have finished assessing the larynx, **withdraw the scope slowly** and **examine the important anatomical structures** once again **in reverse order**. You may often see more clearly or even notice things you may have missed on the way in the first time round.

Offer the patient some **paper tissues** for blowing his/her nose (and hopefully not for wiping away tears!) after the procedure. Pass the scope to your nursing staff for **decontamination**. You can now finish the procedure by **documenting** the findings in the patient's notes and explaining the findings to the patient.

TIps and hints

- Adopt a calm and reassuring manner throughout the procedure. This will automatically put your patient at ease.
- Fully explain what you are going to do to the patient before and during the procedure and inform him/her what he/she should expect to experience.
- Always perform FNE with the patient sitting down or lying 45 degrees semi-recumbent in bed as well as have a nursing staff/colleague present during the procedure. As with all unpleasant procedures (i.e. even with insertion of a venflon!) occasionally the procedure can cause a vaso-vagal episode.
- Give specific instructions to the patient at different stages of the procedure in order to optimise the view you can get from the FNE.
- When withdrawing the scope, remember to let go of the finger lever in order to avoid 'hooking' and traumatising the soft palate and floor of the nasal cavity on the way out.
- In cases where Co-phenylcaine is used, the oropharynx can often be anaesthetised in addition to the nasal cavities. The patient may complain of a lump sensation in his/her throat and that swallowing is difficult. Reassure the patient that this will resolve in 1–2 hours and advise the patient not to eat or drink anything hot in this period incase he/she sustains an oropharyngeal burn.

OSCE checklist

- Dons gloves
- Connects scope to light source
- Holds and operates scope correctly
- Applies lubricating gel (optional)
- Rests scope under tongue
- Explains procedure
- Positions patient correctly
- Visualises anatomical structures
- Completes examination correctly
- Hands patient tissue
- Washes hands
- Thanks patient
- Documents procedure
- Provides postprocedure advice

18 Gynaecological Examination and Cervical Smear

Charlotte Smith and George Goumalatsos
Ptychio Iatrikes

Video Time | 3 mins 38 s

Overview

Gaining proficiency at gynaecological examination can be a daunting aspect of medical training. As if the surreal 'professional vagina' session that most medical schools now run with *real humans* wasn't enough, then there is the OSCE where dropping the speculum on the examiner's foot is something to avoid. Most Foundation Year rotations contain either General Practice or A&E, both of which will expose you to women medically requiring examination of this nature. This simple guide to speculum and bimanual examination, and taking smears and swabs, will give you confidence to safely and proficiently perform a gynaecological examination, and save an angry, overworked and sweating on-call gynaecology registrar from shouting at you down the phone in the middle of the night for referring a patient without examining her properly.

The **smear test** is a very common procedure performed in general practice and gynaecology clinics. Getting the speculum examination right will alleviate most of the discomfort associated with a smear test because the cervix is poorly supplied with sensory nerves. If you perform smears regularly, you will need a Smear Taker Number. This allows the local laboratory to keep an eye on how many successful smears you take (you are only allowed a tiny proportion of them to be 'inadequate'). Smear tests are performed as part of a cervical screening programme in England for instance at regular,

How to Perform Clinical Procedures, First Edition. Matthew Stephenson, Joshua Shur and John Black.
© 2013 John Wiley & Sons, Ltd. Published 2013 by John Wiley & Sons, Ltd.

3-yearly intervals from 25 to 49 years of age, then 5-yearly until 64 years. They are also indicated for unexplained vaginal bleeding or an abnormality seen on speculum examination. **Swabs** (usually high vaginal and endocervical) are best taken during speculum examination and are indicated for vaginal bleeding, vaginal discharge, pelvic pain and suspected pelvic infections. **Bimanual examination** is used to assess uterine size, mobility and pain, as well as evidence of adnexal masses.

Make yourself familiar with the **types of speculums** available in your trust. Fumbling around will not fill the woman, who is lying semi-naked and feeling vulnerable, with confidence. Look confident, even if you are feeling awkward and embarrassed. You are not the one lying with their genitals exposed to a stranger.

There are two types of bivalve (Cusco) speculum:
- **Plastic** clear speculums, which are all-in-one with just a movable 'nut' to fix the blades open. These are **single use** and require **no prior assembly**, therefore the much-feared fumbling is less likely
- **Metal** speculums, which generally have the hinged piece. These require a very small amount of assembly. These are also **cold**. Metal speculums can either be **single or multiple use**

Sims speculums are more commonly used to examine for vaginal prolapse in the left lateral position or in theatre during gynaecological operations. They are generally not used for routine vaginal examinations.

Indications for speculum exam	Contraindications	Complications
• Visualise cervix • Smear test • STI screening • Suspected STI • Unexplained vaginal bleeding • Menorrhagia • Pelvic pain or dyspareunia • Abnormal vaginal discharge • Foreign body, eg retained tampon • Vaginal or cervical mass • Prolapse • Look for signs of miscarriage • Obstetric indications, e.g. threatened preterm labour, antepartum haemorrhage	• Patient refusal • No chaperone available regardless of gender of doctor • No vagina • Be aware that patients who are virgo intacta can find speculum examinations more uncomfortable; you should use an extra small or small speculum and ask your registrar to assist you	• Discomfort • Vaginal bleeding • Patient unable to tolerate procedure

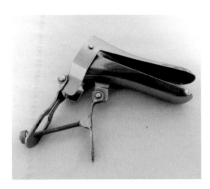

A bivalve speculum (metal)

Procedure

Talk to the woman and **make her feel as comfortable as possible**. Try and distract her – it will make you look more confident and distract you from the nakedness of the situation. It is not only awkward for the woman to have a stranger inserting things in her vagina but for you as well. Involve your **chaperone**. They can help you in making the woman less tense. However, make sure you are not overfamiliar with her. It's a careful and delicate balance.

Make sure you have the **correct patient**, for the **correct procedure**. Check for any **allergies**, and that you have confirmed the **indication;** excluded any **contraindications; explained** the procedure and taken verbal **consent**. Now **wash your hands**! Ensure your **chaperone** is in the room.

Make a mental note of what you are planning to do and gather the appropriate equipment. If you are taking swabs, you need to be sure that they stay sterile until the swab is taken. It is nigh-on impossible to open extra things when your hands are slippery from lubricating jelly. Use your chaperone wisely. Now **assemble everything you need on a trolley**. A sterile drape on the examination bed will do equally well. Everything needs to be clean but not sterile, unless you are taking swabs. Open the speculum packet and don't just squeeze a small amount of jelly onto the blades of the speculum. Use it all, unless you're taking a smear test, in which case too much gel, especially on the tip of the speculum, will interfere with the results. If you are using a metal speculum, try and take the edge off the freezing metal by holding it under warm water (not hot!) or in your gloved hand for a minute or so. Everything you might need is included in the equipment textbox, including for taking a smear test and swabs.

Equipment you need:

- Clean trolley
- A lamp
- Appropriate size of speculum – for most people, medium is adequate
- Lubricating jelly (water-based for smear test)
- Gloves (use sterile gloves for obstetric exams)
- Tissues for the woman to wipe off excess jelly

For a smear test and swabs
- Cytobrush
- Bottle of smear medium
- Plain charcoal swab for taking HVS (usually black packet)
- Swab for taking ECS for chlamydia (viral medium, often pink or orange packet)

Speculum examination

Before you start, ask the woman to empty her bladder if she needs to. Stand to the patient's right, at the level of her hips. If you are left-handed and the bed allows, go to the other side, you are allowed to do this! Make sure the **bed is laid as flat** as the woman is comfortable with. Ask the woman to put her feet together, bend her knees and bring her heels towards her bottom, letting her knees drop apart. Explain to her that she can ask you to stop at any time. **Expose the patient** so the woman's vulva is uncovered and you can clearly see where you are aiming for. This can be more of a problem in the obese, or those with reduced mobility. Asking the woman to place rolled-up hands underneath her buttocks can help. **Switch your lamp on** and shine it on the vulva. Try and angle it slightly so that when you look into the speculum, your head won't block the light out.

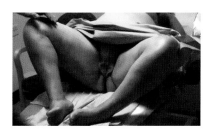

The patient should be positioned with the knees flexed and legs apart

Put on your gloves, and inspect the vulva. Dermatological conditions such as lichen sclerosis, lichen planus, infections such as human papilloma virus (HPV), candida, age related and atrophic changes, scars from previous childbirth or female genital mutilation should be noted and recorded. **Gently part the labia** with your left hand. Expose the vaginal introitus and **insert the lubricated speculum sideways** with your right hand (so the widest diameter is running anterior to posterior and the handle is to one side). You are **aiming forwards and downwards**, towards the sacrum. **Advance the speculum, rotating it so that the handle is now anterior**. You will need to go almost up to the hilt in most people to get to the cervix. **Open the blades slowly**, waiting for the cervix to gradually come into view. When you can see the cervix, you can **fix the blades open** with the nut if you wish. If you can't find the cervix, repeat the above procedure. Sometimes you need to aim more posteriorly or anteriorly, or change for a larger speculum. If you really can't see it, there's no shame in doing a digital examination to feel for where you are aiming.

Check that the cervix looks normal – generally, it should be pink, smooth, regular in outline and with a small os in the middle. If there are any abnormalities present, take note of these and remember to write them down when you have finished the examination.

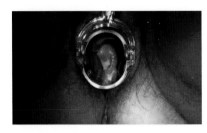

The speculum has been inserted and the cervical os can be visualized

Smear test

If there is vaginal bleeding, you should not take a smear test. Clean the cervix with a cotton wool bud. **Insert the middle of the cytobrush** into the cervical os. **Rotate** clockwise 5 times. Ask your chaperone to take the lid off the smear medium, then remove the brush from the os and **agitate/crush the brush** in the smear medium 10 times. Check that no lumps of anything obvious remain on the brush, remove the brush and close the lid. Set to one side.

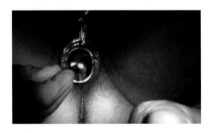

The cytobrush is inserted into the os

Swabs

For a **high vaginal swab**, ask your assistant to **open the swab packet** in a sterile manner, exposing the handle of the swab. Remove from the packet and **insert into the posterior vaginal fornix** (at the back of the cervix) and **rotate** a few times. Remove the swab and insert it straight into the swab medium.

To take an **endocervical swab** (most commonly for chlamydia), again ask your assistant to open the swab packet in a sterile manner. These swabs have a **large cotton bud to clean the cervix** with. Do this first, then **insert the actual swab** into the cervical os and **rotate** a few times. Remove and replace into the special medium.

Removing the speculum
This can be as uncomfortable as inserting it in the first place. This is because the cervix can become trapped between the blades of the speculum on removal. Firstly, **undo the nut** on the speculum handle. **Keeping the blades open, gently pull back on the speculum until you are clear of the cervix**. Now allow the vagina to do all the work in closing the blades for you (this reduces the chance of pinching the vaginal wall between the two blades). If you're planning on doing a bimanual examination, go on to do this now and wait to fill in forms etc until after this is complete.

If you are not planning on doing a bimanual, **dispose of any clinical waste** in the appropriate bin. Now, gather up any swabs and smear bottles, give the woman the tissues and leave her in peace to sort herself out and get dressed. Remember to **document** your examination and findings, **label your swabs** and **fill in the appropriate forms**.

Bimanual vaginal examination

This should be undertaken **after the speculum examination**. This is because a digital vaginal examination could potentially contaminate the vagina with skin flora and alter the results of vaginal swabs. The jelly used to perform this examination could also contaminate a smear test if this were to be taken afterwards.

The purpose of bimanual examination is to determine:

- size of uterus
- mobility of uterus
- relation of the uterus to the cervix (flexion) and to the vagina (version)
- shape and consistency of cervix
- uterine or adnexal masses or tenderness
- evaluate for signs of gynaecological pathology: acute, for example cervical motion tenderness in pelvic inflammatory disease or ruptured ectopic pregnancy and chronic such as endometriotic changes.

Keep the woman in the same position. You are still wearing your gloves, and the only equipment you need is lubricating jelly (note that **you still need your chaperone**). **Squeeze some lubricating jelly** onto the index and third fingers of your right or left hand (depending on your handedness). Gently **part the labia** with your non-lubricated hand and **insert your index finger**, first waiting for the woman to relax. Then **insert your third finger**, again sideways, into the introitus. **Aim** downwards and forwards towards the sacrum, following the contour of the vagina and **rotating** so that your palm is facing upwards by the time you reach the cervix. Be careful to not press on the clitoris or stick your fourth or fifth fingers into the anus.

Place your fingers underneath the cervix, **in the posterior fornix**. With your other hand (use the ulnar edge of your fingers) **palpate the abdomen** from the umbilicus downwards, moving your hand towards the pubic symphysis until you can feel the uterus between your two hands. Make a note of its **size** (often compared to an orange) and **version** (ante- or retroverted). In a retroverted uterus, the fundus is palpable through the posterior fornix. In a normal sized uterus, it will not be palpable until just above the pubic symphysis. In obese patients, it is often extremely difficult, if not impossible! Also make a note of **uterine mobility**. A mobile uterus is normal whilst a fixed one is not (a sign of pelvic adhesions, due to endometriosis, prior pelvic surgery or previous pelvic infections, for example).

Now **move your vaginal hand** to the left lateral fornix, and **move your abdominal hand** to the left lower quadrant. You are trying to feel the left adnexa between your two hands. If normal, you will not be able to feel anything. Make a note of any tenderness. Now **do the same for the right adnexa**.

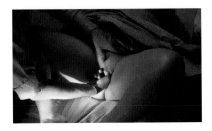
Bimanual examination

Lastly, **check for cervical motion tenderness**. Place your fingers once again in the posterior fornix and tip the cervix on your fingers. The woman will complain of pain if this is present. If pain is limiting the examination from the offset, asking the woman to exhale can aid abdominal muscle relaxation. At the end of the examination, remove your fingers, put your gloves in the appropriate waste bin, leave the woman some tissues and let her get dressed behind the curtain. **Document** your findings and **explain** them to her once she is dressed. If you performed a speculum and took swabs or a smear, remember to **dispose of any associated waste**, **label your specimens** and **fill any required forms** in.

OSCE checklist (speculum and smear)

- Introduces self
- Requests chaperone
- Instructs patient to empty bladder
- Ensures correct positioning
- Lubricates speculum
- Inserts speculum sideways into vagina then rotates
- Opens speculum gently
- Identifies cervix
- Cleans cervix
- Inserts cytobrush into os and rotates 5 times
- Agitates brush in smear medium ten times
- Removes speculum without catching cervix
- Disposes of waste
- Replaces covers on patient
- Labels specimen and fills in appropriate forms
- Documents procedure
- Explains findings

OSCE checklist (bimanual vaginal examination)

- Introduces self
- Asks for a chaperone
- Positions patient correctly
- Inspects external genitalia
- Inserts index and third finger into vagina
- Places fingers in posterior fornix
- Palpates abdominally from umbilicus downwards
- Assesses uterine size
- Places fingers into lateral fornices to assess adnexae
- Assesses for cervical motion tenderness
- Replaces covers on patient
- Disposes of waste
- Documents findings

19 Hand Hygiene

Angeline Boorer

Video Time | 3 mins 20 s

Overview

Healthcare associated infections (HCAI) are localised or systemic conditions that develop as a result of medical interventions or when patients receive treatment in hospitals, nursing homes or even in their own homes. They are one of the **biggest causes of avoidable harm** and unnecessary death associated with healthcare and can affect any part of the body including the urinary system, respiratory system, gastric system and the skin of patients that have had a surgical procedure.

Current prevalence and incidence data helps to inform infection, prevention and control measures, however the true extent is difficult to determine because HCAI can present postdischarge for up to a year. The effect of HCAI is to extend lengths of stay, anxiety to the patient and their relatives and disrepute to the healthcare facility. Risk factors include extremes of age, certain specialties and the complexity of treatment, indwelling devices and poor infection control such as hand hygiene.

The hands of healthcare workers are easily contaminated by micro-organisms after routine contact with the hospital environment, patients or after contact with blood or bodily fluids. The acquired microbes are then readily transferred to patients unless we clean our hands before patient contact. This mode of 'indirect' transmission is typically how Methicillin-resistant *Staphylococcus aureus* (MRSA), norovirus, influenza and to some extent *Clostridium difficile* infection *(CDI)* are transferred. The skin on our hands also harbours commensal, or resident, flora which also pose an infection

How to Perform Clinical Procedures, First Edition. Matthew Stephenson, Joshua Shur and John Black.
© 2013 John Wiley & Sons, Ltd. Published 2013 by John Wiley & Sons, Ltd.

risk to patients particularly during surgical techniques, insertion of indwelling devices and wound care.

Hand hygiene (HH) is the physical removal (or killing) of micro-organisms and is known to be the single most effective measure for the prevention of cross infection. Hand hygiene may be performed using (a) **liquid soap and water;** (b) **alcohol-based gel** (AHG) or **hand rub;** or (c) **antiseptic hand wash**. The method chosen depends upon the episode of care, the available resources and to an extent personal preference.

Washing hands with soap and water will remove transient micro-organisms and render the hands socially clean. This level of decontamination is sufficient for general social contact and some clinical care activities.

AHG provides a practical alternative to hand washing providing the hands are not visibly soiled and is more effective in reducing the bacterial load of the hands due to its ability to destroy both resident and transient skin flora on the hands.

National strategies to improve HH include the clean**your**hands (CYH) campaign implemented to reduce HCAI particularly MRSA blood stream infections and CDI. An element of the CYH campaign is that AHG should be situated at the 'point of care' namely the patient's bedside.

The **World Health Organization** (WHO) have developed a concept known as '**Your 5 Moments for Hand Hygiene**' which is universally accepted in healthcare, rationalising when and why hands should be cleaned to reduce the risk of HCAI. This principle is also helpful in dispelling myths and modifies needless hand hygiene practice predisposing to hand irritation.

This concept is also widely supported by patient groups and regulatory bodies because HCAI are also thought of as a **patient safety** issue, and a marker for quality care. The **five moment concept** is illustrated in this section.

The five moments must be applied at all times regardless of the healthcare setting. Whether in the patient's own home, operating department, outpatients, or specialist departments such as NICU, ICU and CCU.

Each 'moment' describes when and why hand hygiene (HH) must be performed.

Moment 1 Before patient contact. This will protect the patient from becoming colonised or infected by microbes on our hands. If our hands are visibly clean using the AHG at the 'point of care' is recommended.

Moment 2 Before an aseptic task. This 'moment' is critical in preventing micro-organisms from entering the patient during an aseptic procedure such as inserting or manipulating an indwelling devices such as PVC, CVC, Urinary catheters, NG and ET tubes or wounds. HH should be performed as close to the site of care as possible, avoiding recontamination with objects such as the patient's curtains, their

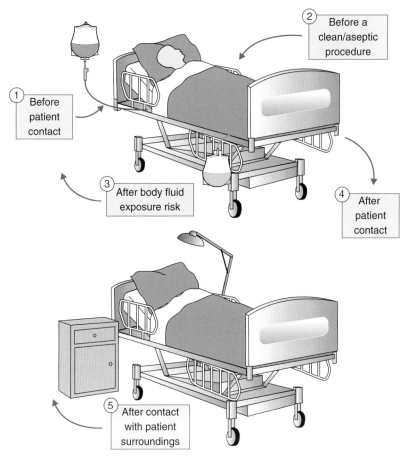

Based on WHO poster 'Your 5 Moments for Hand Hygiene' (Reproduced with permission of WHO)

environment or their own skin or gown. Soap and water followed by AHG is required for this moment OR a hand wash using an antiseptic liquid soap.

Moment 3 After contact with body fluid exposure risk. HCWs are also at risk of infection by potentially infectious body fluids, blood and respiratory secretions from patients. HH must be performed immediately after contact with body fluids even if the hands are visibly clean and when gloves have been used. Soap and water is recommended but AHG can also be used.

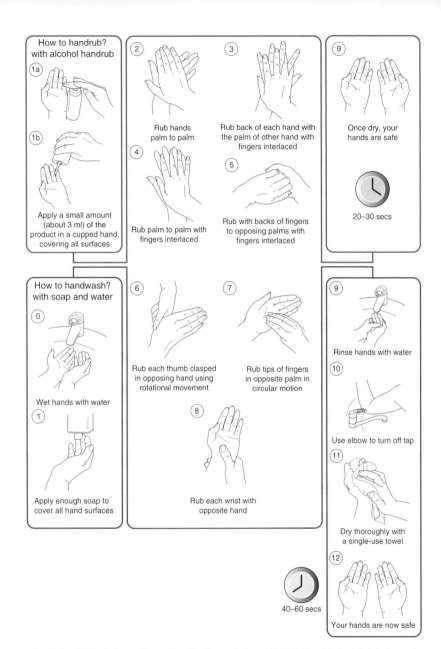

Hand cleaning techniques. (Reproduced with permission of NHS National Patient Safety Agency)

Moment 4 After patient contact (if leaving the patient zone). This will reduce the dissemination of the patients' flora to the HCW, environment and other patients and HCW.

Moment 5 After contact with the patient's surroundings (if leaving the patient zone). The patients' immediate zone may be colonised with their flora. The hands of HCWs may become contaminated by their flora without touching the patient.

Procedure

An effective hand washing technique involves three stages, (i) **preparation,** (ii) **washing and rinsing**, (iii) **drying.**

HCW should already be 'bare below the elbows', not wearing any bracelets or watches. A plain wedding band/partnership ring is acceptable. In the video we demonstrate the effects of handwashing with your sleeves rolled down and wearing a watch and ring. Any cuts and abrasions on the hands must be covered with a waterproof dressing.

The following procedure demonstrates how to carry out effective hand decontamination using soap and water, alcohol hand gel and using an antiseptic hand wash.

Effective hand washing: step-by-step procedure

Action	Rationale
Wet hands under tepid running water	Wetting hands begins the cleaning process by removing loose dirt and micro-organisms. It also prepares the hands to receive the soap solution and facilitates lathering. Wetting hands prior to soap is thought to reduce skin irritation. Running water is preferred as a water-filled sink can re-contaminate the hands. Tepid water is more comfortable for the HCW, and is thought to produce more lather. Cold water may cause discomfort. Hot water is not recommended due to the damaging effects on the skin
Apply foam or liquid soap to the palm of the hands	Excessive soap may lead to skin damage. Applying soap to the palm will help distribute the soap product evenly to the rest of the hands and remove dead skin cells and transient pathogens present on the hands

(Continued)

Effective hand washing: step-by-step procedure (*cont.*)

Action	Rationale
Vigorously rub the hands systematically together. The suggested methodology is: • Rub palm to palm x 5 times • To reach the interdigital spaces of the hands rub the fingers of one hand over the dorsum of the other hand and interlace the fingers • Repeat the procedure on the palmer side of the hands to reach the palmer interdigital area • Rub the back of the fingers across the palm of the other hand with the fingers interlocked • Clean the fingertips by rotating them in the palm of the other hand • To clean the base of the thumb, clasp it in the palm of the other hand and rotate the thumb • Finally clean the wrist by clasping it in the other hand and rotate the wrist • Each sequence should be repeated on both hands. This should take approx. 20 seconds	Vigorously rubbing hands promotes the removal of dead skin cells, and transient pathogens and dirt. It is also thought to reduce skin irritation Using a systematic technique will clean all the surfaces of the hands, focusing upon areas that are frequently missed such as between the fingers, back of the hands and thumbs
Rinse hands thoroughly with running tepid water	Removes all traces of soap, surface skin cells, pathogens and dirt
Dry hands using disposable paper towels – pat until thoroughly dry	Disposable paper towels are preferred over communal towels which can re-contaminate clean hands. The drying patting action removes transient pathogens, protects the skin from damage caused by friction
Turn taps off using the elbows or clean paper towels	Prevent re-contamination of hands from micro-organisms which may be on the taps.
Discard paper towels in the appropriate (or recycling) waste stream. If these options are unavailable, use the clinical waste stream	Use foot operated waste bins, avoid touching the lid as this will re-contaminate the hands

Procedure for using Alcohol Hand Gel (AHG)

Action	Rationale
Apply 1–3 pumps of AHG to visibly clean hands.	Adequate AHG must be used to allow time to cover all the surfaces of the hands before product evaporates.
AHG should be vigorously rubbed in all the surfaces of the hands using the 7 steps until the product has fully evaporated	Rubbing vigorously reduces risk of skin damage. AHG destroys transient and resident bacteria as it evaporates.
The HCW may wish to wash their hands with liquid soap and water following several applications of the AHG	To remove build-up of emollient

Procedure for aseptic hand decontamination

There are two recommended methods to achieve aseptic hand decontamination:

Action	Rationale
1. Using liquid soap and water as per 7 stage technique then dry hands Proceed to apply AHG	Liquid soap and water will remove dirt and debris from the hands allowing maximum effectiveness of the AHG disinfection. The application of AHG will destroy resident skin flora reducing the risk of infection when handling indwelling devices or wounds
2. Using 4% Chlorhexidine gluconate and water as per 7 stage technique then dry hands	Antiseptic solution will remove both resident and transient micro-organisms from hands.

Procedure for using hand moisturiser

Action	Rationale
Apply a small amount of hand moisturiser to all the surfaces of the hands and rub until absorbed	Small amount of the moisturiser will be more rapidly absorbed.
Its use is recommended three to four times a day and is of greatest benefit when the moisturiser has time to sink into the dermis. Recommend used when leaving the clinical area for breaks and at the end of the day	To work effectively, i.e. repair the skin mantle and replace natural oils lost through hand hygiene. Ideally the HM should be left on the hands for a minimum of 20 minutes
Communal jars of emollients are not recommended in clinical areas as they could easily become contaminated and cause cross-infection	The palm of the hands do not contain pores therefore HM is of most benefit when applied on the backs of the hands, fingers, thumbs and wrists
Hand cream is contraindication Following an antiseptic hand wash. Prior to donning gloves in preparation for an aseptic procedure	Over use can cause blocked pores, and impede the efficacy of subsequent AHG and the antiseptic hand wash

Glove usage

Gloves do not replace the need to perform HH and when an indication for HH occurs during glove usage, the HCW must remove the gloves, perform HH and don another pair of gloves if still indicated.

HH must always be performed following the removal of gloves because hands may become contaminated during removal and gloves may have tiny perforations affecting their integrity. Gloves are single use items and should never be decontaminated with alcohol since this will lead to holes and leakage of soap and water.

Looking after our hands

Correct HH techniques (wetting hands before applying soap, thorough rinsing, drying hands by patting with disposable paper towel) reduces skin damage. Counter-intuitively, the vigorous application of soap products and AHG is associated with less skin irritation. When the skin is damaged it becomes more heavily colonised than healthy intact skin and presents a risk to the HCW and the patient. The use of moisturiser which is readily available in clinical areas is also encouraged (see above).

Hand decontamination for patients

Patients must have the opportunity to clean their hands whenever they wish to. This is to be encouraged following toileting and before and after eating or handling food.

Definitions

Alcohol Hand Gel (AHG) or alcohol hand rub

An alcohol containing preparation (liquid, rinse, gel or foam) designed for application to the hands to kill micro-organisms. AHG should not be used when caring for patients with diarrhoeal illnesses.

The Five Moments

The critical moments during a patient's care when staff clean their hands to prevent the transmission of microbes that can cause HCAI.

Hand hygiene (HH)

A general term to denote hand cleansing using either alcohol hand rub, soap and running water, or, antimicrobial soap and running water. This procedure is to be understood and consistently practiced by all HCWs to decrease the incidence of HCAI.

Hand hygiene opportunity

When one of the 'Five Moments' are encountered and HH is practised.

Hand washing

Washing hands with plain or antimicrobial soap and running water.

Healthcare Associated Infection(s) (HCAI)

A localised or systemic condition that was not present or incubating at the time of admission unless the infection was related to an admission involving another healthcare facility.

Non-compliance

Failure to perform hand hygiene in accordance with the Five Moments.

Patient zone

The patient and their immediate surroundings.

Point of care

The place where three elements come together: The patient, the HCW and care or treatment involving contact with the patient or his / her surroundings. Alcohol hand rub must be accessible within arms reach of where patient care or treatment is taking place.

Resident flora

Micro-organisms occupy a particular body site and are part of the normal flora. They are usually beneficial but can cause infections if they get into another body site, for example, the normal skin flora from the hands if they enter the blood stream. They reside under the superficial cells of the stratum corneum and are also found on the surface of the skin.

Transient flora

Micro-organisms that colonise the body for a short duration (hours/weeks) of time. The bacteria are easily 'picked up' from contact with people, objects and environmental surfaces. They colonise the superficial layers of the skin and are more amenable to be removed by routine hand washing.

Visibly soiled hands

Hands on which dirt or body fluids are readily visible.

OSCE checklist

- Rinses hands with warm water
- Applies soap solution to palm
- Rubs palm to palm
- Rubs backs of hands
- Interlaces fingers
- Rubs backs of the fingers with opposite palm
- Rotates around thumbs
- Rubs finger tips to palm
- Rubs wrists
- Rinses hands and turns off taps
- Dries hands correctly

20 Intramuscular Injection

Emma Stewart-Parker

Video Time | 2 mins 9 s

Overview

Let's imagine you're the F1 on call… It's 3 am. You've hit a quiet spell and decide to take a well-earned siesta in the mess. The on call bleep sounds and it's one of the nurses and they inform you that a patient on the ward isn't looking too well. After discarding the remains of your dinner in the bin, you inform them you're on your way.

On your arrival, your nursing colleague informs you the patient is looking increasingly confused and, whilst reeling off their observations, announces that the patient has a BM of 1.2. That'll be the culprit…

You're led to a drowsy patient, ventilating themselves but clearly unable to swallow. In this situation, oral glucose just won't do.

The best thing would be to insert an intravenous cannula, and give a bolus of 50 mls of 50% glucose. That would definitely do the trick. Unfortunately the patient has no veins to speak of. Time is running out. What are you going to do now?

You remember – 1 mg intramuscular injection of Glucagon! And this is your get out of jail card. It will buy you the time needed to secure intravenous access and set about the broader work of dealing with hypoglycaemic emergencies.

This may be a lengthy aside from IM injections but it's a handy reminder. Far more commonly the IM route is used for the drugs listed in the following textbox. By far the most commonly administered class of drugs given by this route (worldwide) has to be immunisations. Although usually administered by trained nursing staff, intramuscular

How to Perform Clinical Procedures, First Edition. Matthew Stephenson, Joshua Shur and John Black.
© 2013 John Wiley & Sons, Ltd. Published 2013 by John Wiley & Sons, Ltd.

injections offer a handy route and you should have an understanding of how to perform the procedure.

Intramuscular injection is the administration of a drug directly into the muscular layer of tissue deep to the subcutaneous plane (skin and fat). The benefits of this route include a potentially faster absorption rate as unsurprisingly, muscle given its relative physiology and function tends to have a far meatier vasculature than the subcutaneous layer. Absorption rates will also depend on their individual pharmacological properties.

Indications	Contraindications	Complications

• Certain drugs:
  ◦ Adrenaline
  ◦ Glucagon
  ◦ Vaccinations
  ◦ Antibiotics
  ◦ Analgesia
  ◦ Antiemetics
  ◦ Naloxone
	• Coagulopathy (can cause very painful muscle haematomas), e.g. patient on warfarin
	• Allergy (to intended drug)
		• Haematoma
		• Cellulitis

Procedure

Make sure you have the **correct patient**, for the **correct procedure**. Check for any **allergies**, and that you have confirmed the **indication;** excluded any **contraindications; explained** the procedure and taken **consent**. Now **wash your hands**!

Assemble all of your equipment on a trolley away from the patient. You will need everything in the equipment textbox.

Acceptable **injection sites** include the upper outer quadrant of either buttock and the outer aspect of the upper arm or thigh. It's worth noting that the intramuscular injection is deeper than the subcutaneous one, and the volumes injected are usually larger. They are

Equipment you need (on a sterile tray/trolley)

- Green needles (21G) x 2 (one for drawing up, the other for injecting)
- Syringe
- Non-sterile gloves
- Alcohol based wipe
- Drug to be injected
- Diluent (if intended drug requires it)
- A plaster/cotton wool

generally **more painful** as the muscle fibres separate to accommodate the delivered drug. In light of the increased volumes, the commonest site is the buttock, simply because the gluteal muscles are large and more accommodating.

Check the drug with a colleague – The five R's offers a useful model before administration:

- Right **drug**
- Right **dose**
- Right **route**
- Right **patient**
- Right **date and time** of administration.

Finally, check the **expiry date** of the drug. Never give an out of date drug.

Wash your hands and don your **gloves**. **Inspect** for any obviously damaged areas of the overlying skin at the intended injection site, such as burns, areas of cellulitis, infection or eczema. Avoid previous injection sites where possible. **Clean the skin** with the alcohol preparation using concentric circles outward from the site of intended puncture. Allow it to dry completely before proceeding.

Carefully **open the vial**. Plastic vials are easy – a small pull and twisting action should do the trick. Do take particular care with glass vials – you are at risk of a nasty glass-related injury – which whilst not serious is painful enough to forever make you wince at the sheer sight of a glass vial. Break the neck of the vial over the site indicated by a small dot on the neck (which is a manufactured area of weakness) and you should hear a 'pop' as the glass goes. You may want to hold the vial with a swab to protect your fingers from it.

Draw up your drug and any diluents (if needed) using one of the green needles. Once completed, **discard the empty vial** (including the vial top) directly into a sharps bin if it's glass. **Expel any air** in the syringe or drug before **discarding the needle in a sharps bin**. Double check the prescription is correct, and the details of the chart match the patient's wrist band, confirming this information verbally as a final check. Make a final check of allergy status.

De-sheath the needle, and gently **pinch up** the area for injection with your non-needle holding hand (take care not to contaminate the puncture site) at a **90° angle**. Warn the patient of an **impending scratch** and **insert the needle** all the way down into the muscle – this is usually achieved by advancing around two-thirds of the way down the needle (again this will vary depending on how well padded with adiposity the patient may be). Once you're happy with the positioning, **aspirate back on the syringe** to check you have not inadvertently entered a large vessel. **Slowly expel the contents** of the syringe until empty. This again may vary from drug to drug, but if you inject too quickly, you will

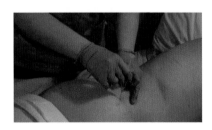

The needle inserted into the upper outer quadrant of the buttock at 90° to skin

cause pain as you spread the muscle fibres rapidly. By injecting in a more controlled manner, the fibres spread less abruptly.

After the drug has been administered, **withdraw the needle** and **dispose of your sharps immediately**. Apply a piece of gauze should any bleeding ensue, and a gentle massage can help disperse the drug and ease the pain. A plaster can be placed over the puncture site if so desired.

Remember to **sign, time and date the prescription chart** and complete any necessary **documentation**. **Thank the patient and wash your hands**.

OSCE checklist

- Assembles equipment correctly
- Checks patient details, allergies and drug chart
- Positions patient correctly
- Checks drug with 2nd member of staff
- Draws up medication and expels air
- Disposes of ampoule
- Changes needle
- Inserts needle at appropriate angle
- Aspirates needle
- Injects medication
- Removes needle and massages injection site
- Disposes of sharps immediately
- Washes hands
- Thanks patient
- Documents procedure
- Provides postprocedure advice

21 Intravenous Fluid Infusion

Eric Lindberg

Video Time | 5 mins 10 s

Overview

In the main, intravenous fluids are given by nursing staff to patients, however there will be many situations, particularly in emergencies, when you need to be able to set up an IV line yourself and administer IV fluids. It's really very easy and there's no reason not to master it.

One could write a whole tome on fluid balance and IV infusions but the whys and wherefores of choosing how much fluid to give and what kinds of fluid to give, are beyond the scope of this book. What this chapter does provide, however, is a whistle-stop tour of commonly administered fluids, the lines and giving sets used, fluid pumps and a succinct demonstration of **how to safely prime a line and give an IV infusion**. Hopefully this will help to clear those muddy waters, making things clear as a bag of saline.

The word 'intravenous' literally means 'within a vein', hence intravenous infusion or therapy refers to the delivery of a liquid substance directly into your designated patient's vein. Fluids are by far the commonest substances delivered via this route. Often, this is in an attempt to correct a volume deficit or electrolyte imbalance. Intravenous routes can also be used for administration of medications. For example, saline may act as a diluent or solvent for a particular medication requiring reconstitution. Intravenous nutrition is also available for those patients requiring parenteral feeding in the form of TPN, although this must be given into a large central vein. Blood (see above, Chapter 9: Blood Transfusion) is given intravenously, along with cytotoxics and chemotherapy. Due to previous

How to Perform Clinical Procedures, First Edition. Matthew Stephenson, Joshua Shur and John Black.
© 2013 John Wiley & Sons, Ltd. Published 2013 by John Wiley & Sons, Ltd.

mishaps, it's worth noting that chemotherapy can only be administered by trained professionals on a designated, usually oncological ward.

Indications	Contraindications	Complications
• Fluid depletion (dehydration) • Haemorrhage • Electrolyte disturbance • Decreased fluid intake • Excessive outputs: stoma, drains, diarrhoea, vomiting • Fluid balance discrepancy	• Hepatic impairment (caution with lactate containing fluids) • Hypo/hyper natraemia/ kalaemia • Congestive cardiac failure • Chronic kidney disease (RRT) • Fluid retention	• Fluid overload • Electrolyte disturbance (particularly Na^+ and K^+) • Pulmonary oedema • Peripheral oedema

Procedure

Make sure you have the **correct patient**, for the **correct procedure**. Check for any **allergies**, and that you have confirmed the **indication;** excluded any **contraindications; explained** the procedure and taken **consent**. Now **wash your hands!**

Assemble all of your equipment on a trolley away from the patient. You will need everything in the equipment textbox. Ensure you have the correct volume of fluid, and any additional prescriptions to be added. It's worth getting a useful colleague to check any additional electrolytes/prescriptions to be added to the infusion for optimal patient safety.

Wash your hands and **put on your apron and gloves. Draw up a saline flush** (5–10 mls) using a green needle and syringe, in preparation. This is to flush your line prior to commencing any infusion and check the intravenous device is

Equipment you need (on a sterile tray/trolley)

- Disposable apron
- Non-sterile gloves
- A sited, patent intravenous cannula or other intravascular device
- A green needle
- 10 ml syringe
- Saline flush
- Alcohol based wipe
- Fluid to be administered as prescribed
- Giving set: normal line/dual chamber filtered (for blood)
- Fluid pump (if precise delivery required) and appropriate giving set
- Drip stand
- Fluid balance chart

patent. Once you have drawn up the flush, **dispose of your sharp safely**.

Before you approach your patient, **check the fluid** to be infused is within use by date, and that the packaging is intact. The same applies to your giving set. Carefully remove the fluid from its packaging, and inspect it. There should be no sediment or foreign bodies visible.

Unwrap your giving set, and check its integrity. Proximally, there will be a spike (which is plunged into the port on the fluid bag) closely followed by a chamber and distally, a connector which can attach to the cannula. The roller ball clamp can be rolled to occlude the line when slid proximally. **Set the roller ball clamp to 'closed'** to avoid spillage of the fluid. **Twist off the plastic cap** at the insertion port on the IV fluid bag, and **hold the fluid upright** with your non-dominant hand.

Using your dominant hand, **depress the chamber to expel air**, and **plunge the spike** into the insertion port, fully inserting it into the fluid. **Release the chamber** and **invert the bag** of fluid. The chamber will fill under the vacuum you have created by compressing the chamber. **Allow the chamber to fill** to the level mark. Fluid should advance down the line towards the roller ball

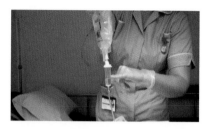
The fluid chamber being filled

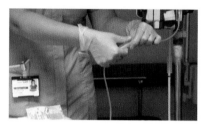
This is the roller ball clamp which you open and close with your thumb

clamp (which should be closed). Continue to slowly prime your line by **gradually opening the roller ball clamp**. Watch the line as it fills distally for any air bubbles. If air bubbles are apparent, these must be run out at the end of the line before the infusion can be initiated.

Once a column of fluid (free of bubbles) reaches the protective sterile cap, **close the roller ball clamp**. You have now primed the line. Check again the patient's allergy status verbally and that this correlates with the drug chart. Ensure the fluids to be given are as prescribed, and cross check the patient's identifiers using the wrist band and the drug chart. This should also be verified verbally.

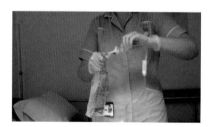
The spike on the end of the giving set is about to be pushed into the bag

Open your alcohol-based swab, and **clean the port on the patient's cannula**. Once it has had time to dry, **flush** the cannula using 5 mls of normal saline. This should be pain-free and inject easily. There should be no swelling or surrounding tissue distension as the flush is injected. Remove the protective cap and **attach the connectors together** using a screw-like rotatory action. **Slowly open the roller ball clamp**, and **set the drip to the desired rate** by slowly adjusting the roller ball accordingly. Once you have established the desired rate of infusion, **hang the fluids** on the drip stand.

Make sure that any fluids given are **signed, timed and dated** with clear notation of the rate of infusion. Once the intravenous infusion is complete, **close the roller ball clamp** and **unscrew the connector**. **Clean the intravenous ports** with an alcohol wipe and **dispose of the clinical waste** accordingly. Ensure to maintain an accurate fluid balance chart, carefully documenting all fluid input against the total output.

Other ways of giving IV fluids
Fluid pumps
Fluid pumps vary in appearance based on manufacturer, but essentially they all work on similar principles; they infuse a set volume over a specific time. This means that an accurate rate of infusion can be delivered to patients who require careful fluid management.

A specialised giving set is required if you wish to infuse via means of a fluid pump. The line contains a section that runs through the pump, and this is usually made from silicone. The silicone section of the line sits inside the pump. Exactly the same technique is used for priming the line as above, all bar one amendment. The silicone section of the line has an increased potential for air bubbles to form and adhere to it.

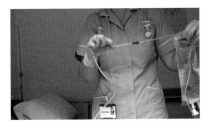

The compressible silicone section of the line which is then lined up with the coloured markers in the machine

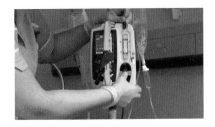

Prime the line using the same method as described above. When fluid reaches the silicone component, fill

this section horizontally allowing fluid to travel up the silicone strip against gravity. This reduces the risk of air bubbles congregating at this section of the giving set. Once the fluid appears past the silicone, fill the remains of the line as usual. Close the roller ball clamp once the air free column reaches the protective cap.

Turn on your pump and check that it's fully functional. Open the door and slot the flanges at either end of the silicone section into the designated retainers. They should mount with a convincing click! Close the door to the pump and screw the connectors together (obviously after cleaning and flushing the intravenous device).

Use the electronic keypad to set the volume to be infused, followed by the rate. For example, a 500 ml two-hourly bag will run at 250 mls per hour. Once the rate has been set, press 'start' to commence the infusion. There is a locking system to stop the infusion if necessary.

Rapid infuser devices

Finally, in the emergency setting when aggressive fluid therapy is required, a rapid infuser can be used. This device allows volumes to be administered at the fastest rate possible. The device is very simple, and consists of a pouch which holds the bag of fluid to be given. The pouch is in fact an inflatable bladder attached to a manual pump and pressure gauge, which can be inflated manually using a pump action.

A large bore intravenous device is required for rapid delivery – usually a grey or an orange gauge is acceptable. Prime the line as if you were using a standard giving set. Pass the bag of fluid into the bladder, and secure it by passing the loop through the perforation at the top of the fluid bag. Hang the rapid infuser on the drip stand and open the roller ball clamp once you have connected the line to the intravenous device. Proceed to inflate the bladder by pumping the handle. As the bladder inflates, the fluid is put under pressure, which can be monitored using the pressure gauge built into the

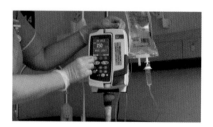

The pump switched on and set to 250 mls per hour

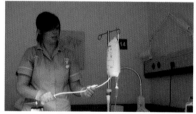

The fluid within the rapid infuser pouch which is being inflated

rapid infuser. Note a continuous stream through the chamber as opposed to a 'drip'. Note that you will need to increase the pressure by further inflating the bladder as the volume decreases in the fluid bag to maintain the rate of delivery.

OSCE checklist

- Dons apron and gloves
- Draws up saline flush
- Checks expiry date
- Disposes of sharp
- Checks IV fluids
- Checks allergy status
- Closes roller ball clamp on line
- Inserts tip of line into fluid bag with chamber depressed
- Releases chamber to fill
- Primes line correctly
- Closes roller ball clamp and checks for air bubbles
- Hangs fluids
- Cleans port
- Flushes port with saline
- Connects line
- Opens clamp and sets rate of infusion
- Records details in drug chart correctly
- Washes hands
- Thanks patient

22 Intravenous Injection

Video Time | 2 mins 25 s

Overview

As hinted at in the introduction to this book, older consultants today experienced a very different F1 experience (or Houseman year as it was then known) to the one we have today. There were no phlebotomists and few nurses had training in intravenous cannula insertion. But that's not all, it was the job of the Houseman to prepare and give all of the intravenous medications! Can you imagine? As well as everything else you have to do! This is one of the (many) reasons older consultants often have little sympathy for juniors today claiming they're overworked. Anyway, we digress. Being able to prepare and give intravenous medications is still a vital core skill for any doctor. In primary care you're likely to still do it on home visits for example. Some drugs also are still not given by some nurses, for example IV morphine and sometimes radiological contrast.

Intravenous injection refers to the process of giving a medication directly into the patient's vein. Administration of an IV injection may involve giving the medication rapidly as an IV push or bolus directly from a syringe, intermittently over a set period of time using an IV secondary line, or continual delivery of the medication mixed with, for example, a bag of fluid. IV medications are most often administered through a peripheral line or cannula, but they can also be given via others means, such as a central line, an implantable port or peripherally inserted central catheter (PICC).

The primary purpose of giving an IV injection is the potential to initiate a rapid systemic response to said medication: For example, during cardiac arrest, adrenaline is given as part of a protocol and the drug is immediately available to the patient providing a peak serum concentration in seconds. This particular method of

How to Perform Clinical Procedures, First Edition. Matthew Stephenson, Joshua Shur and John Black.
© 2013 John Wiley & Sons, Ltd. Published 2013 by John Wiley & Sons, Ltd.

administration is by far the fastest way to deliver a drug. It bypasses the digestive enzymes associated with oral delivery and the liver or 'first pass metabolism'. It also avoids the poor absorption rates and often discomfort associated with the other parenteral routes: Subcutaneous and intramuscular.

For these same reasons it can make this route more dangerous. For example administering a penicillin based antibiotic to a penicillin allergic patient intravenously will precipitate a much more severe reaction than if given orally.

Drug delivery rate is an important factor associated with IV injection. Some medications are designed to be delivered quickly over the course of seconds or a few minutes to obtain the desired therapeutic effect, whilst others are given more slowly over the course of hours or even a day(s). Each drug delivery rate is different, so refer to pharmaceutical guidelines or your local trust protocol in order to achieve the desired effect.

For the purpose of this chapter, we shall look at giving a routine IV injection which has been reconstituted from its powdered form (IV Co-Amoxiclav).

Remember that extravasation of some drugs can cause tissue necrosis so be alert to this. Ensure that the drug is administered intravenously and not via an artery - if you are administering the drug yourself always double check where the line is going.

Indications	Contraindications	Complications
• Rapid delivery of drug • Administration of IV medication • Emergency - where rapid delivery of drugs is required • Titration of drugs, e.g. insulin, analgesia • Medication that cannot be administered by any other route, e.g. inotropes	• Allergy to drug • Occluded peripheral line • Preexisting phlebitis • When alternative routes would be as effective • Arteriovenous fistula (avoid insertion of peripheral line required for IV injection)	• Allergic reaction (to drug) • Pain • Infection • Phlebitis • Crystalisation of drug and vessel occlusion • Tissue irritation and oedema • Air embolism • Medication error

Procedure

Make sure you have the **correct patient**, for the **correct procedure**. Check for any **allergies**, and that you have confirmed the **indication;** excluded any **contraindi-** **cations; explained** the procedure and taken **consent**. Now **wash your hands!**

Assemble all of your equipment on a trolley away from the patient. You will need everything in the equipment textbox.

IV drugs are often stored on the ward in a powdered form, which obviously you can't inject. Therefore, the drug has to be reconstituted or combined with a diluent to form a solution in preparation for injection, with the commonest diluents being saline or water for injection (a distilled sterile form). This is the case with intravenous co-amoxiclav.

The drug is normally carefully labelled complete with instructions detailing:

- The name of the drug
- How much diluent you will need to add (mls)
- What type of diluent you must use
- The total resulting volume following reconstitution (this is more than the volume of diluent used as the drug itself occupies a certain volume)
- The concentration of the resulting volume (mg/ml)
- The expiry time post reconstitution

It's definitely worth reading the label thoroughly. Sometimes the reconstitution volumes differ for specific routes of injection (i.e. IV vs IM) for the same drug. A little bit of reading will prevent a woopsie. Also pay attention to the fluid suggested and follow the instructions clearly. IV drugs may not be compatible with certain IV fluids or other drugs. Drug incompatibility is a real risk to the patient, as this may evoke a precipitation reaction causing crystalisation, which will at least block the IV line and at worst inflict an embolus effect on the patient, spelling trouble.

The reconstitution should take place away from the patient's bedside. A treatment room is ideal. **Wash your hands** and put on a pair of **non-sterile gloves**. Attach the green or blue needle to a 20 ml syringe. **Desheath** the needle taking care not to inadvertently stick yourself. After **checking the expiry date** and other details of the drug as described above, draw up the volume of diluent required for reconstitution as specified in the drug data sheet. **Expel any air** from your syringe.

Remove the plastic cap of the powdered drug and **clean the rubber top** with an alcohol-based wipe. **Insert the needle** into the bottle, piercing through the rubber top. **Slowly inject** the volume of the syringe into the bottle containing the drug in its powdered form, whilst simultaneously making gentle circular motions with the bottle to assist mixing of the drug with the liquid. Make sure the entire volume of diluent is combined with the drug.

Since you have injected liquid into a closed container, the **pressure** inside the bottle (which now contains the dissolved powder) will have **increased**. Once you're happy that the powder has dissolved, **invert the bottle** and **release the pressure** you have been applying to the syringe plunger. You will see the reconstituted drug begin to fill the syringe independently under its own pressure. As the syringe nears filling and the bottle is almost empty, **aspirate on the syringe** to assist with the last few drops. Remove the syringe from the bottle and **dispose of the sharp**. If the bottle is made from glass, this will also need to go in the sharps bin. It's good practice to check your reconstitution with a helpful colleague. Cap the syringe.

Happy days! You are now ready to administer the IV injection. **Draw up 10 mls of saline flush** before taking a trolley with everything you need to the patient's bedside. Check that the drug has been **correctly prescribed**, and that the intended injection isn't a drug sensitivity of the intended patient. **Confirm patient identifiers** correspond to the drug chart and the patient's identity

band. Check this information verbally. Ideally the patient should have had a cannula sited in preparation.

Wash your hands again and change your non sterile gloves. **Swab the port** connected to the cannula with an alcohol wipe and allow this to dry. In the meantime, **expel any air** from the syringe containing the intended injectables. **Open the clamp** on the port of the cannula, and **flush with 5 mls of saline**. It should flush easily and not cause any discomfort.

Once you're happy with the integrity of the peripheral line, **connect the syringe** containing the drug to the connector – this is normally achieved using a screwing action, as most trusts use the Luerlock variety. **Slowly inject the drug** over the time period suggested by the manufacturer's guidelines – in the case of co-amoxiclav, this is 5–7 minutes. **Observe the patient** as the drug is administered. If they display any signs of allergy, stop injecting. The injection should be pain free. Observe the arm for any swelling or discolouration – this could

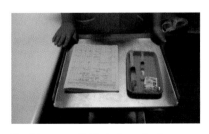

The things you will take to the patient's bedside: The drug chart, a saline flush, the drug for injection and an alcohol wipe

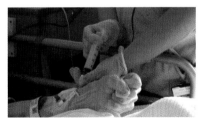

The syringe with the drug in it is connected to the connector port, and the drug injected

indicate the cannula has tissued and it will need re-siting. There are no prizes for filling the fascial compartments of the forearm!

Once you have finished injecting, **disconnect the syringe** from the connector, and flush the line with the remaining 5 mls of saline flush. This ensures that every ounce of drug has entered the patient's circulation and isn't still sitting in the cannula. **Close the clamp**, and **wipe the port clean** with a second alcohol wipe. You're almost done. **Discard any sharps** and dispose of any clinical waste appropriately. Remember to **sign, time and date** the prescription properly.

OSCE checklist

- Assembles equipment correctly
- Dons gloves
- Cleans top of vial
- Draws up sterile water
- Reconstitutes drug with correct amount of water
- Replaces needle with bung
- Disposes of sharps immediately
- Confirms correct patient identity, prescription and allergies
- Cleans cannula connector port
- Flushes line
- Administers drug over correct timescale
- Flushes line
- Cleans connector
- Signs drug chart
- Washes hands
- Thanks patient

23 Large Bore Chest Drain

Joy Edlin and Michael Marrinan

Video Time | 6 mins 10 s

Overview

Inserting a large bore chest drain is often considered one of the most exciting procedures to learn as a junior. Picture yourself in A&E, the trauma bleep goes off, a patient is rolled in with multiple injuries. Right sided rib fractures and a haemopneumothorax. The patient's beginning to struggle for breath. In you swagger, put down your Starbucks coffee and deftly pop a tube in to the right pleural cavity. The patient's lung refills, his breathing improves and you receive a Christmas card each year for life. If only that was how it usually goes …

In reality, large bore chest drains are wonderful things – and in the right hands they are truly lifesaving. But it's been said that there isn't an organ in the body that hasn't been pierced by one at one time or another. If you're going to learn to put chest drains in, which you should, learn to do it well. But of course, that's why you're reading this book.

Remember there are two kinds of chest drain, the one described in this chapter, the **large bore chest drain**, and the other one, the **Seldinger chest drain**. For more details on the differences, see below, Chapter 34: Seldinger Chest Drain.

Procedure

Make sure you have the **correct patient**, for the **correct procedure**. Check for any **allergies**, and that you have confirmed the **indication;** excluded any **contraindications**; **explained** the procedure and taken **consent**, which in some trusts needs to be in the written form for a chest drain. Now **wash your hands**!

How to Perform Clinical Procedures, First Edition. Matthew Stephenson, Joshua Shur and John Black.
© 2013 John Wiley & Sons, Ltd. Published 2013 by John Wiley & Sons, Ltd.

Indications	Contraindications	Complications

• Hydrothorax
• Haemothorax
• Pneumothorax
• Hydropneumothorax
• Haemopneumothorax
• Postoperatively (always placed prophylactically during thoracic surgery)
	• Refractory coagulopathy
	• Infection in overlying skin/ soft tissues
	• Lung densely adherent to chest wall
	• Relative contraindications:
	  ◦ Loculated effusion
	  ◦ Pleural scarring (thickening)
	  ◦ Presence of diaphragmatic hernia
	  ◦ ->likely to require drainage under ultrasound or CT guidance or surgically
		• Pneumothorax/tension pneumothorax
		• Haemothorax
		• Bleeding
		• Infection
		• Injury to solid organs

Assemble all of your equipment on a sterile trolley away from the patient. You will need everything in the equipment textbox. Make sure you have an **assistant** throughout, they will need to hand you things as you will be sterile, and they will also need to connect the drain to the drainage bottle.

Set up the **equipment trolley** and **prepare your closed drainage system** with the underwater seal. The latter is formed by adding sterile water to your collection bottle up to the premarked line. This creates a one-way valve, which allows air out of the pleural space, but prevents air getting in.

Ensure radiographic images are available. It's now **mandatory to have three-dimensional imaging** of the chest before chest drain insertion in the form of either a **CT or ultrasound** (yes we know that's 2D, but as soon as you move the probe around it gives you a 3D understanding), except in dire emergencies.

Examine the patient. This will help you confirm the indication and side, and identify the necessary **anatomical landmarks** as well as help demarcate the **fluid or air level**.

Your anatomical landmarks are:
• **5th intercostal space** (ICS)
• **Anterior axillary line** (immediately lateral to the lateral border of pectoralis major)
• The literature quotes the **safe triangle of insertion** as bordered by the lateral side of the pectoralis major muscle anteriorly, the anterior border of latissimus dorsi posteriorly, the axilla apically and a

Equipment you need (on a sterile tray/trolley)

- 'Your' equipment
  - Face mask
  - Sterile gown
  - Sterile gloves
  - Surgical hat to cover hair
- Procedure equipment
  - Dressing pack or chest drain insertion pack which includes:
    - Sterile cover for trolley
    - Gauze swabs
    - Gallipot or tub for skin cleaning solution
  - Chest drain, usually 24–30F
  - Sterile drapes
  - Skin cleaning solution (e.g. Betadine)
  - Connecting tubing
  - Closed drainage system allowing underwater seal
  - Sterile water
  - Local anaesthetic (10–20ml 1% lidocaine)
  - 10ml syringe
  - Green (21G) needle
  - Blue (23G) needle
  - Scalpel
  - Robert's artery forceps or similar
  - Suture, e.g. 1 silk with large curved needle
  - Sterile scissors
  - Occlusive dressings

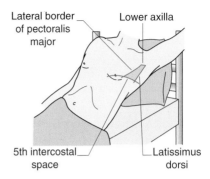

The safe triangle

How do I identify the 5th ICS?

From the **Angle of Louis**, the palpable junction between the manubrium and the sternum, you can palpate laterally into the 2nd ICS. From here you can 'walk' your fingertips counting down to the 5th ICS.

You may occasionally place the drain in an ICS above this, the 4th ICS is OK, but in other ICSs *only* if detailed imaging (CT) is available and *only* if considered very carefully and after discussion with a senior. In these cases it must almost certainly be inserted under ultrasound guidance. Remember that important neurovascular structures and intra-abdominal organs may be damaged (even fatally) if the drain is inappropriately placed.

Why must I place the intercostal drain along the anterior axillary line?

This ensures that you **avoid the midaxillary line**. This is important because the **long thoracic nerve** runs here and damage to this can cause winging of the scapula.

Placing the drain in this line also avoids damage to breast tissue, avoids having to dissect through the muscular pectoralis major and avoids unsightly scarring should the drain be placed more medially.

line along the 5th ICS/through the nipple inferiorly. These borders should be viewed with caution as the anterior border of latissimus dorsi actually lies behind the midaxillary line and you *must* insert the drain anterior to the midaxillary line.

Inserting a large bore chest drain can be pretty uncomfortable even after infiltration with local anaesthetic, consider giving **premedication** in the form of benzodiazepines or opioids. In a trauma patient, also consider giving **prophy-lactic antibiotics** depending on the extent and mode of injury.

Position the patient **resting at 45°** with the arm on the affected side raised over their head. This allows you free access to the site and stretches the chest wall, opening up the rib spaces.

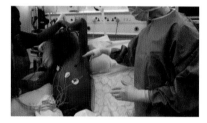

Positioning to stretch out the chest wall

Identify your anatomical landmarks again and **mark the site** where you deem it safe to insert the drain.

Now you can **scrub** and **don your sterile protective clothing**. **Clean** the site with skin preparation. **Drape** the patient, leaving only the site and its immediate surroundings exposed. An aperture drape is ideal for this as it has a hole in the middle, which can be aligned with the planned drainage site.

Prepare to **infiltrate local anaesthetic** (LA) into the site. When inserting the needle, aim for the top of the 6th rib, but before you hit it deviate upwards slightly, so that the **needle rests on top of the rib**. This avoids damage to the intercostal neurovascular bundle. Gently pass the needle through the tissues, whilst applying

constant negative pressure on the syringe, until you enter the pleura. If you're able to easily **aspirate** fluid or air (depending on the indication) into your syringe you know it's safe to proceed at this position. If you're unable to aspirate fluid or air it's unsafe for you to place the drain here. You should then **ask for help** from a more senior member of your team. If you're experienced, however, you may attempt to insert the drain in a higher ICS instead. If in any doubt, chest drains are better placed under ultrasound guidance.

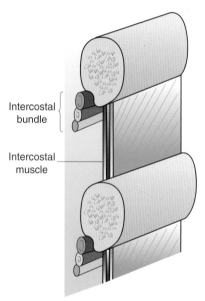

Intercostal bundle

Intercostal muscle

Intercostal bundle on the undersurface of the rib

Once positive aspiration has confirmed a safe drain position, **infiltrate the**

tissues generously with LA. Leave this to work its magic for a couple of minutes. Confirm that the tissues are numb before you **make a small incision** (2–4 cm depending on level of experience) in the skin using the blade. The incision shouldn't be much wider than the tube diameter. Perform a **blunt dissection with your index finger/s**, and carefully with the tip of the forceps if required, pass through the tissues aiming for the rib before you deviate **on top of the rib**. Note that this is effectively done blindly by touch alone, you can't see the dissection. Continue the blunt dissection through the intercostal muscles until you reach the pleura.

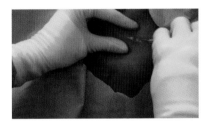

A stab incision through the skin only

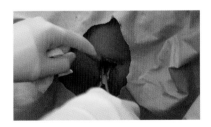

Blunt dissection using tips of the forceps

Keep your tract patent with the index finger from your non-dissecting hand.

Otherwise the tract is easily lost and the dissection made more difficult.

Pierce the pleura using blunt dissection. The pleura can sometimes be a little tough, in which case you may pierce the pleura with the *tip* of the forceps *only*. Make sure you hold your fingers 1-1.5 cm from the tip of the forceps so that no more of the instrument can be advanced and cause damage. **Never** use the stiff metallic trocar, which often accompanies the drain. This was once used all the time but is now deemed unsafe, too many atria were damaged in the making of this advice. It can however come in handy in the garden when **planting seeds**.

Breaching of the pleura will cause an **immediate release** of air in the case of a pneumothorax or immediate release of blood or fluid in the case of a haemo- or hydrothorax, respectively.

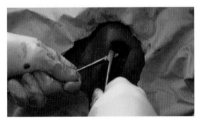

The pleura has been pierced and blood is pouring out

Enlarge the pleural opening with your finger/forceps and perform a **pleural sweep** with your finger to ensure that lung is not stuck to the pleura.

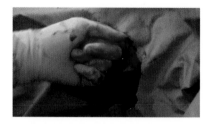

The index finger is performing a sweep around the inside of the pleural cavity to ensure there are no adhesions to it

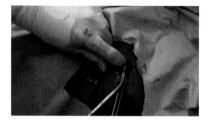

The chest tube is mounted on the forceps to aid initial passage

Insert the chest drain. It can help to mount it on artery forceps just to get through the passage you've created in the chest wall. Aim it apically for a pneumothorax or for a hydropneumothorax or haemopneumothorax, in other words whenever there's air to drain. In the latter cases, the fluid will still eventually drain when the patient is lying down. For hydro- or haemothoraces aim the drain infero-posteriorly. If the patient is on **positive pressure ventilation**, suspend ventilation briefly during insertion of the tube and remember to ask for ventilation to be resumed immediately after drain insertion

and before securing the drain. Insert the drain to **at least 10–12 cm**.

You have inserted a large drain, which may allow free passage of air into the pleural cavity (potentially creating a tension pneumothorax) or hoses pleural contents out onto your shoes. So, **without letting go of the drain**, with one hand, kink or clamp the drain temporarily and immediately connect it to the underwater seal via the connecting tubing to avoid the above. To the other end of the tubing must be attached, the chest drain bottle. Your assistant will do this bit. If you had to clamp the drain during this bit, take it off now. Remember to **maintain the depth** of the drain in the chest cavity throughout this process, that is, don't let the drain come out or push further in than you wanted.

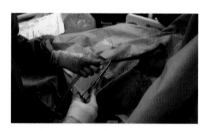

The chest drain has been connected to the tubing which is connected to the chest drain bottle, the clamp is about to be released

You then need to put in at least three different sutures for three different reasons, something strong like 1 Silk will do the job for all of these. First you need to secure the drain in place with a **stay suture**. Take a bite of the skin

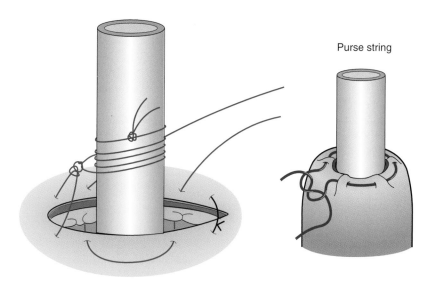

Purse string

The red suture is the stay suture holding the drain in place. The green suture is the horizontal mattress suture. The black suture is the interrupted suture to narrow the wound around the drain. Note, on the right is a purse string suture (blue) - do not use these for drains

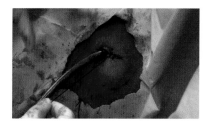

The sutures in place. The ends of the horizontal mattress suture are being pulled gently just to demonstrate that they're left untied

either side of the wound and then tie a loose knot, then wrap it several times around the drain tube and tie it. Secondly you may need to insert at least one interrupted suture to narrow

the wound around the chest tube to ensure it's airtight. Thirdly you *must* also place a **horizontal mattress suture** (not a purse string suture). This is a suture that you insert through the skin but don't tie down, you leave the ends long. When it's time for the drain to be removed you can pull on the ends to close the hole left by the drain. Don't place a suture through the drain!

If you're treating a pneumothorax you must place the drain on **negative suction** (-2 kPa to -5 kPa). This will immediately cause air to bubble through the water seal.

If you're treating a haemothorax in the trauma context, keep a close eye on haemodynamics (your patient should also have two wide-bore IV cannulae as part of the ATLS protocol) and on the volume of blood drained. If 1500 ml blood is immediately drained early thoracotomy is likely to be required.

Clean and dress the site and **arrange a chest X-ray** to monitor the pneumo- or hydrothorax and the position of the drain. If the chest X-ray reveals a new pneumothorax, the drain should be placed on negative suction to aid removal of the air and re-expansion of the lung.

Dispose of your sharps directly into a sharps bin and your waste into a clinical waste bin. **Wash your hands** and **record the procedure** clearly in the patient notes.

OSCE checklist

- Checks three-dimensional imaging
- Identifies the chest wall landmarks
- Identifies site for drain in 4th or 5th intercostal space
- Scrubs and dons appropriate sterile personal protective attire
- Assembles equipment correctly
- Positions patient appropriately
- Preps the skin
- Creates sterile field
- Reconfirms position for drain placement
- Warns about a 'sharp scratch'
- Raises a bleb of local anaesthetic under the skin
- Infiltrates local anaesthetic into deep layers
- Tests the effect of the local anaesthetic
- Makes an incision in the line of the rib space
- Bluntly dissects through chest wall
- Opens pleural lining bluntly
- Sweeps finger around inside of chest wall
- Passes chest drain tip into chest cavity mounted on clip
- Secures tube with silk stitch
- Temporarily clamps or pinches tube to prevent excess leakage
- If indicated, takes sample of pleural fluid to send to the lab
- Attaches tubing to chest drain bottle
- Attaches drain to tubing
- Inserts horizontal mattress suture
- Applies occlusive padded dressing
- Requests a chest x-ray
- Washes hands
- Thanks patient
- Disposes of sharps and waste
- Documents procedure
- Provides postprocedure advice

24 Large Bore Chest Drain Removal

Video Time | 1 min 41 s

Overview

Congratulations! You have successfully performed your tube thoracostomy, skillfully placing that plastic tubing into the thoracic cavity to remove air or fluid from the pleural space. You've *even* managed to avoid those vital structures which would otherwise have made for an unpleasant day for the patient, yourself and the legal department. Now, maybe a few days later, it's time to take it out.

Drain removal time is governed by both the initial indication and the patient's response to the therapy. It might be the next day, it might be 5 days later. Essentially, as with any drain, **it comes out when it's finished doing its job**. This is confirmed by the following **clinical parameters**:

1 No more **bubbling** – which would indicate there's no more air to come out
2 Little or no **fluid draining** – which would indicate there's no more fluid to come out
3 Return of a more **normal chest examination**, for example clear lung bases (although there may be some residual crackliness after an effusion)

Also if the drain has stopped swinging (more accurately 'swinging of the drain' means a rise and fall in the fluid level in the tube within the drainage bottle on inspiration and expiration, the drain itself doesn't physically swing!) this indicates the tip of the drain is no longer well placed within the pleural cavity which means it's probably blocked, or that the pleura is adherent to the tip, and entirely useless.

Nevertheless, **always get a chest x-ray before removal** to confirm that all the air and/or fluid has indeed gone, otherwise it may for example be more appropriate to try

How to Perform Clinical Procedures, First Edition. Matthew Stephenson, Joshua Shur and John Black.
© 2013 John Wiley & Sons, Ltd. Published 2013 by John Wiley & Sons, Ltd.

and **reposition the drain**. So in other words chest drain removal requires both clinical and radiological checks beforehand.

Drains should not remain in situ for longer than absolutely required. Remember you have breached the skin at the point of entrance, thus increasing the risk of **infection** via the insertion site as time progresses. It's time to remove that potential vector before the patient's natural skin flora (potentially including some MRSA nasty's!) have a party in the pleural cavity.

Unfortunately for you, unlike removing a Seldinger chest drain, it's not quite as simple as just cutting the drain stay suture and yanking it out. Drain removal method plays a crucial factor in the patient's recovery. The ideal aim of drain removal involves removing the tube, whilst simultaneously preventing air getting into the pleural cavity landing you back at square one. It's a bit like opening the back door without letting the cat out. It does require some thought and a simple appreciation of respiratory physiology. Providing you follow the advice here, this procedure is very, very simple.

The debate about whether to remove the drain during the inspiratory or expiratory phase rages on, however there is in fact a right way of doing it, and this is supported by the **British Thoracic Society**. Theoretically, during inspiration the lungs are at full expansion and therefore it can be argued that there will be little space for air to enter the pleural cavity. Conversely, during full expansion of the lungs, a negative intra pleural pressure is established, potentially leading to entrainment of air into the pleural cavity when the drain is removed generating a pneumothorax. Alternatively if you remove the drain during expiration this creates a positive pressure in the pleural space, also stopping any air getting in. The problem here though is – what happens when you suddenly cause someone pain in their thoracic wall? They suddenly breathe in, sucking in that air. However there is a third way, and fortunately, it's the right way. The **Valsalva manoeuvre**. Ask the patient to strain in your preferred Valsalva way (e.g. close your mouth and hold your nostrils closed with one hand and try to blow your nose

Indications	Contraindications	Complications
• No further air draining (for pneumothorax) • No further fluid draining (for effusion/haemothorax) • No longer swinging • Clinical findings confirmed on x-ray	• Incomplete resolution of the primary indication	• Pneumothorax • Haemothorax • Bleeding

until your ears pop, or whatever). This not only creates a positive pleural pressure but is also distracting to that pain reflex of sudden inspiration.

Procedure

Make sure you have the **correct patient**, for the **correct procedure**. Check for any **allergies**, and that you have confirmed the **indication** (clinically and radiologically); excluded any **contraindications; explained** the procedure and taken **consent**. Now **wash your hands**!

Assemble all of your equipment on a trolley away from the patient. You will need everything in the equipment textbox.

Equipment you need (on a sterile tray/trolley)

- Gloves
- Scissors
- Sterile gauze
- Adhesive op-site dressing
  If there's no horizontal mattress suture already in place:
- Suture kit containing:
  o Needle holder
  o Forceps
  o Scissors
- Some skin prep
- Local anaesthetic, e.g. 1% lidocaine
- A syringe
- A green needle (21G)
- A blue (23G) needle
- A suture, e.g. 2–0 Nylon

With the patient **positioned upright** sitting towards the edge of the bed, carefully **peel off the dressing** exposing the drain and the sutures. You may be faced by a confusing bunch of bits of thread

matted around the drain. Decipher what's going on. There will be at least one suture tied around the drain – this is the stay suture, you'll need to cut this to take the drain out. There may be one or two interrupted sutures just going through skin which have been tied together and have been used to narrow the wound around the tube. Finally, depending on the kindness, or quality of the clinician who inserted the drain, they have hopefully also left either a **purse string** or **mattress suture** (we would hope specifically it's the latter) precisely which depends on how they put it in. From here on in it shall be referred to as the **purse string/mattress suture** to cover both possibilities. This is a suture inserted into the skin but the ends are not tied, they're left loose so that when pulled, the wound closes, without the need for the malarkey of putting in another suture when the drain comes out. So once the dressing is off, look carefully at the suture(s) present to check for this.

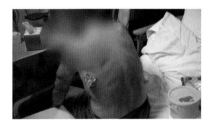

The patient is sat up and leaning forward, this gives the appearance in this picture that the drain is sited more posteriorly than it should

Insertion of a horizontal mattress suture for
later wound closure

Purse string

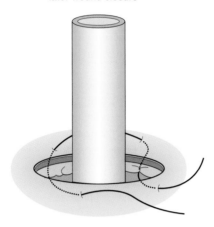
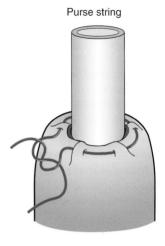

Difference between horizontal mattress suture and purse string suture, remember for when you're
putting one in, the latter is not advised

If your colleague hasn't done this now's the time to **put in your own horizontal mattress suture** (no deep sutures are required), never put in a purse string suture. **Prep** the skin, infiltrate some **local anaesthetic** to the area and **insert the suture** in the manner illustrated in this section. A 2-0 nylon suture for example, would be fine. Make sure you are prepared beforehand with the relevant kit on your trolley, or at least that it's close to hand so you can get it when you discover said problem when you take the dressing off. Make a note of whoever put the drain in so that you can suitably punish them when you next see them.

Explain to the patient what you're about to do and **give clear verbal instructions with regards to the Valsalva manoeuvre**. Ask the patient to clarify what you have told them, and practise if necessary before you cut the sutures securing the drain.

Carefully **cut the stay suture(s)**, not the purse string/mattress suture! Ask the patient to make their **Valsalva effort**. With a swift action, **pull the chest drain out** in one movement whilst **simultaneously pulling on the ends of the purse string/ mattress suture**. Gently at first, then firmly once the drain pops out. If you have an assistant, one person can pull on the drain and the other person on the suture. The skin should come together as soon as the drain comes out. **Tie the ends** of the purse string/mattress suture ensuring that the edges of the site are adequately apposed. You need an **airtight seal**.

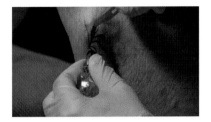

The upper suture, that is also tied around the tube is cut with the suture cutter. You can see the ends of the horizontal mattress suture below the drain

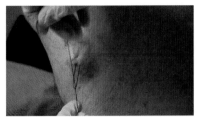

Tie the ends of the horizontal mattress suture together to appose the skin edges

Cover the wound with a transparent **adhesive dressing**. Offer some **oral analgesia** if the patient has any residual discomfort. **Wash your hands** and **discard of any sharps** appropriately if you had to use any and dispose of the chest drain in the clinical waste bin. **Reassess your patient** via means of clinical examination, and perform a set of observations. You must request a **postchest drain removal chest x-ray** to exclude any unintentional injury or recurrence of the pneumothorax. The suture can be removed from the drain site in a week. Finally **document** it all in the patient's notes.

OSCE checklist

- Assembles equipment correctly
- Positions patient correctly
- Removes dressing
- Cuts correct suture
- Instructs patient to perform Valsalva manouvre
- Simultaneously removes drain and pulls on closing suture
- Securely ties suture
- Applies dressing
- Washes hands
- Thanks patient
- Disposes of sharps and waste
- Documents procedure
- Provides postprocedure advice
- Requests a repeat chest x-ray

25 Local Anaesthetic Infiltration

Video Time | 2 mins 10 s

Overview

So you've found a fancy procedure you're keen to do and there's someone willing to supervise you. You're going to put in a chest drain, suture a wound, insert an ascitic drain, etc. There's one thing in common for all of these procedures – one of the first steps is administering local anaesthetic to numb the area. Your chances of doing the rest of the procedure rely on you (a) providing adequate pain relief for the patient, and (b) showing your supervising senior you have the skills to do the simpler steps of the procedure.

You need to know how much of which local anaesthetic drug to give, not only for procedures done purely under local anaesthetic but also as an adjunct during a general anaesthetic (if you numb the surgical field before cutting, you reduce the amount of systemic analgesia the anaesthetist has to give, and the patient wakes up in less pain).

Don't forget, local anaesthetics don't work well in inflamed, infected areas as these are acidotic. Local anaesthetics are weak alkalis and only diffuse through the cell membrane in their unionised (unprotonated) form. If there's a bunch of protons hanging around, as obviously there are in acidic environments, the local becomes ionised and can't cross the membrane. Also, the higher tissue vascularity carries the injected local away quicker.

Local anaesthetics are divided into **esters** and **amides**, examples of the former being benzocaine and cocaine, which are infrequently used. Amides are far commoner, the commonest being **lidocaine** and **bupivacaine**, with or without added adrenaline. The adrenaline locally vasoconstricts and stops the local getting away so quickly, so you can use more of it and its effects last longer. Don't forget that you can

How to Perform Clinical Procedures, First Edition. Matthew Stephenson, Joshua Shur and John Black.
© 2013 John Wiley & Sons, Ltd. Published 2013 by John Wiley & Sons, Ltd.

never use adrenaline on the extremities, for example for a ring block as it can render the extremity ischaemic. Bear in mind that these amide local anaesthetics are metabolised by the liver so their half-lives may be far longer in someone with liver failure; you may want to be sparing with it. Lidocaine's onset of action is quicker and will last one to two hours, whereas bupivacaine will last three to four hours.

Quite frustratingly, if you want to look up how much local you can safely give you'll find many sources giving different concentrations per kilogram (body weight). The following is a safe guideline:

Lidocaine	4 mg/kg
Lidocaine with adrenaline	7 mg/kg
Bupivacaine	2 mg/kg
Bupivacaine with adrenaline	3 mg/kg

Now for some very complicated maths:

In 1 ml of 1% local anaesthetic
  there is… 10 mg of local anaesthetic.
In 1 ml of 0.5% local anaesthetic
  there is…. 5 mg of local anaesthetic.
In 1 ml of 2% local anaesthetic
  there is… 20 mg of local anaesthetic etc.

Example 1

You want to use some 1% concentration plain lidocaine on a 70 kg patient.

Maximum allowed = 70 (kg) × 4 (mg/kg) = 280 mg.
Total volume allowed = 280/10 = 28 ml of 1% lignocaine.

Example 2

You want to use some 0.5% concentration plain bupivacaine on a 50 kg patient.

Maximum allowed = 50 (kg) × 2 (mg/kg) = 100 mg.
Total volume allowed = 100/5 = 20 ml of 0.5% bupivacaine.

Don't give too much! Do this calculation for each patient before you start drawing anything up. Bupivacaine is particularly cardiotoxic with a narrower therapeutic window. The first warning signs are circumoral tingling or numbness, lightheadedness and tinnitus. This can then progress on to tonic-clonic convulsions, coma, respiratory arrest or cardiac arrest, and that would be pretty terrifying if someone's just come in for excision of their mole.

The antidote

If you're using local anaesthetics you must know what to do if you inadvertently give too much and cause cardiac dysrhythmias or worse, a cardiac arrest. Aside from the obvious: stop injecting it and attend to the basic ABCs of resuscitation, the magic drug you must demand is intralipid. Give 1000 ml of 20% intralipid IV in incremental amounts while resuscitating the patient.

Indications	Contraindications	Complications
• To provide an anaesthetised field to proceed with a procedure	• Local infection (as it won't work, see later) • Allergy (rare)	• Cardiac toxicity • Allergic reaction (rare)

Procedure

Make sure you have the **correct patient**, for the **correct procedure**. Check for any **allergies**, and that you have confirmed the **indication;** excluded any **contraindications; explained** the procedure and taken **consent**. Now **wash your hands**!

Assemble all of your equipment on a trolley away from the patient. You will need everything in the equipment textbox.

Equipment you need (on a sterile tray/trolley)

- Green (21G) needle
- Blue (23G) needle
- Syringe
- The local anaesthetic
- Something to clean the skin
- Sharps bin
- The other equipment needed for whatever procedure you're planning

---

Make sure that you have **calculated beforehand how much local** you're allowed to give based on the patient's weight. **Check the local anaesthetic** ensuring it's the correct drug, correct concentration and in date. Open your local anaesthetic agent (if it's a glass vial take care to break it away from the dot on the neck, and try not to cut your fingers on the glass which is very painful).

Wash your hands and **don your sterile gloves**. **Attach the needle** to the syringe. **Desheath** the needle and **draw up** the local from the vial. If your anaesthetic agent doesn't come sterile packed have your assistant open it and hold it upside down, note how it doesn't spill, this is magic (surface tension of the water). Insert the needle into the vial and draw up the required dose of local anaesthetic. Remove the needle and **dispose of it** in a sharps bin. Hold the syringe upright, draw back on the plunger, **tap the syringe**

gently to move bubbles to the top of the syringe and **expel the air**. Place the narrower gauge needle (blue, 23G) that you will use for injection onto the syringe.

To ensure you don't need to practise your Advance Life Support skills do a final check with the patient and their corresponding drug chart for any **allergies**. As the prescriber and the person administering the drug you are responsible. Do bear in mind though that allergy to local anaesthetics is extremely rare.

Clean the area you plan to anaesthetise with your hospital's preferred skin cleaning solution. Unsheath the blue needle and take the syringe in your dominant hand. **Warn** the patient of an **imminent scratch and burning sensation**. The pain of local anaesthetic injection comes from two things: (1) the needle prick (minor); (2) the burning feeling of the local going in (significant!).

There are two broad possibilities for where you want your local to go, and it may be a combination of both: **superficial** (skin and subcutaneous tissues) and **deep**.

Superficial

Bevel up, slowly **introduce the needle** through the skin into the subcutaneous plane. Insert the needle at a **fairly shallow angle**, that is, so it's nearly parallel with the skin. Insert the needle in the **subcutaneous plane** in the desired direction so that the needle is almost completely under the skin, and you can make out the impression of the needle tip – in

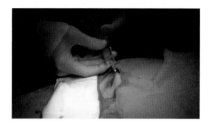

The needle is inserted into the skin edge all the way and then is withdrawn whilst steadily injecting

other words, don't point the needle deeply, and always be able to make out the impression of the needle under the skin. There should be very little resistance to advancement of the needle, if there is you're probably too superficial and are advancing intradermally. Slowly **push down on the syringe plunger** as you equally slowly withdraw the needle, do this all the way until the needle is nearly out of the skin. You will hear people talking about aspirating first, then injecting. This is fine and should be done when injecting deeply (see later), but in the skin you only have tiny vessels, the chance of the needle tip passing through a vein as you withdraw is infintessimally small and even if it does, only an infintessimal amount of local will go into it.

If it's a large area you plan to anaesthetise then you will need to work your way around the perimeter of your operative field injecting the local anaesthetic as you go. Each time you reinsert the needle, go back into an area you have already numbed so that at least the patient won't feel the pinprick.

Deep

For instance you might be inserting a chest drain and you need to anaesthetise the tissues all the way down to the pleura. In this case insert the needle tip just under the skin and inject a small amount of local, this is called, '**raising a bleb**'. Now direct the needle whichever way you want your anaesthetised track and advance the needle. Aspirate gently on the syringe as you advance, checking you do not draw back any blood. Should you aspirate blood you may be in a vessel so reposition the needle. Proceed to infuse the anaesthetic at a steady rate into the tissue plane.

Once you've administered the local anaesthetic remove the needle and **dispose of your sharp immediately into a sharps bin**. You may see a little ooze of blood or local from the puncture site/s, just gently press on this with some sterile gauze. **Wait** for a couple of minutes for the local anaesthetic to work. Prior to starting the procedure **test** that the area is sufficiently anaesthetised. This can be done by using a needle to prick the area. The patient may still feel pressure, pulling and dragging at the site. But if your anaesthetic has worked they should not feel pain.

Dispose of any clinical waste and ensure your **sharps are safely disposed of** in a sharps bin. Finally, remember to **document** everything you've done.

After showing your superb skills off you should have now instilled confidence in your supervisor to allow you to proceed to do the procedure you have set out to perform.

OSCE checklist

- Assembles equipment correctly
- Checks the drug and expiry date
- Attaches needle to syring
- Draws up medication aseptically
- Expels air from syringe
- Changes needle
- Warns about a 'sharp scratch'
- Inserts needle at appropriate angle
- Aspirates
- Infiltrates tissues in correct plane
- Washes hands
- Thanks patient
- Disposes of sharps and waste
- Documents procedure
- Provides postprocedure advice

26 Lumbar Puncture

Video Time | 4 mins 32 s

Overview

This is a procedure to pass a needle between a patient's lumbar vertebrae into the spinal canal to sample (and sometimes drain) cerebrospinal fluid (CSF). You will no doubt have met colleagues rejoicing at managing to obtain a 'champagne tap' from an obese patient, untainted by not even the merest red blood cell. Comments like these manage to elevate the procedure into near mythical status. However there is no hocus-pocus involved in the 'LP', but yes it can be on occasion tricky and a little uncomfortable for the patient. In the main however it really isn't too difficult and with practice anyone can get the hang of it.

Before we go into the details of the procedure it's worth just thinking about the overarching picture. Essentially you will be passing a spinal needle into the sterile subarachnoid space containing CSF. Imagining this is useful as it immediately brings at least three possible complications to mind, which you should consider before performing the procedure:

1 Infection
2 Bleeding
3 Coning

Infection is a particular risk because the CSF circulates throughout the central nervous system and as we all know meningitis can be fatal.

A **bleed** into the CSF can be serious and fatal too. Therefore contraindication for a LP is a severe bleeding diathesis, coagulation disorder or if the patient is on anticoagulation therapy. As you can imagine a non-compressible bleed can go unnoticed for a while and may require surgery to stop. Every

How to Perform Clinical Procedures, First Edition. Matthew Stephenson, Joshua Shur and John Black.
© 2013 John Wiley & Sons, Ltd. Published 2013 by John Wiley & Sons, Ltd.

patient has to have their FBC, INR, and PT measured before attempting a lumbar puncture.

Coning is also extremely serious. Let's imagine a patient with raised intracranial pressure. Now let's imagine suddenly removing fluid from the base of the spine. The induced pressure gradient and net downward force will cause the medulla oblongata, brainstem, midbrain and cerebellum to be squeezed first against the internal structures within the skull (for example the tentorium) and eventually through the foramen magnum itself. As the brain is squashed, the patient's pupils dilate and their eyes point 'down and out' as the third nerve is compressed. Their conscious level will drop and they may develop a hemiparesis and decorticate posturing and eventually their breathing will become irregular and they may die. Telephone your medical defence society. This was avoidable.

However, saying all that the most common complication one might expect is a headache.

The most common indication for an LP is to check for CNS infection (e.g. meningitis). After that an LP is used to assess for any evidence of subarachnoid haemorrhage (SAH). Other diagnostic tests will be to look for any evidence of demyelination (e.g. oligoclonal bands in multiple sclerosis). It can be both diagnostic and therapeutic for example in idiopathic intracranial hypertension. It also helps in diagnosing Guillian-Barre syndrome (GBS), Creutzfeld-Jacobs disease (CJD) and can even help support the diagnosis of Alzheimer's disease and other degenerative diseases. The list is growing…

Head CT

As the consequences of coning are so severe, all patients must be assessed for signs of raised ICP before performing the LP. In the 'good ol' days' this would be with some proper clinical acumen and thorough examination. Any signs of papilloedema would be quickly picked up upon. Nowadays technology has gifted us with a quick, painless and usually accurate diagnostic tool: the spiral CT. Any patient with suspected raised ICP can be whisked into the scanner and a few minutes later the radiologist (and you) will be able to look for tell-tale signs of raised ICP: oedema, squashed sulci or perhaps a great big mass sitting there. This therefore raises the question: who should be CT'd? Obviously there will be some patients with an extremely low pretest probability of raised ICP and in these cases needlessly irradiating a patient is probably not in their best interests. Keeping in mind that papilloedema is a **late** sign, there will also be patients with raised ICP who may be asymptomatic. There may also be patients where you cannot see the optic disc clearly. So what to do? As a rule of thumb patients with no signs of raised ICP (decreased conscious level, no focal neurology or papilloedema) do not require CT. If you cannot see the disc and there is no other reason to suspect raised ICP: again you can perform the LP. What is certain however is that in suspected bacterial meningitis: CT or LP should **NEVER** delay giving antibiotics. If in doubt about whether to CT or not to CT, ask a senior. However in practice nowadays virtually everyone has a CT before their lumbar puncture.

Indications	Contraindications	Complications
Diagnostic • Suspected meningitis/ encephalitis • To assess for SAH • Other diagnostic indications, e.g. in MS, GBS, CJD Therapeutic • e.g. Idiopathic intracranial hypertension	• Local infection at the site of puncture • Raised ICP • Coagulopathy (uncorrected) • Spinal trauma • Congenital lumbar spine defects e.g spina bifida	• Post Dural Puncture Headache (PDPH) (common, up to 20%) • Bleeding • Infection • Pain • Haematoma • Nerve damage • Coning

Procedure

Make sure you have the **correct patient**, for the **correct procedure**. Check for any **allergies**, and that you have confirmed the **indication;** excluded any **contraindications; explained** the procedure and taken **consent**. Now **wash your hands**!

Assemble all of your equipment on a sterile trolley away from the patient. You will need everything in the equipment textbox. Next find yourself a good chair.

Equipment you need (on a sterile tray/trolley)

• Spinal needle
• Sterile gauze
• Manometer
• Sterile cleaning solution
• Local anaesthetic
• Green (21G) and blue (23G) needle
• Syringe
• Three specimen bottles labeled 1 to 3
• Glucose bottle
• Sterile gloves

How not to put your needle into the spinal cord

When doing this procedure one clearly doesn't want to place a needle through the actual spinal cord. We manage this by remembering some basic anatomy. In normal adults, the spinal cord ends at the L1/L2 vertebral body junction at which point it gives off the cauda equina which radiates downwards. By therefore ensuring we enter below this junction then we will avoid the cord 'proper' and at the very worst tickle the cauda equina which is mobile enough to move out of the way. This explains the shooting sensation in their legs that some people experience. There is a handy surface landmark which is a line joining the posterior superior aspect of the iliac crests. This corresponds to L4 or the L4/L5 vertebral junction-bingo! The procedure we describe in this chapter is therefore for adults, and not children where the anatomical landmarks are different.

You need to be seated to do this procedure. Finally find yourself a willing assistant as having someone to open and pass you the specimen bottles makes things so much easier. Finally before you get started make sure to **label the specimen bottles 1, 2 and 3**.

Now you have your equipment **get your patient properly positioned**. Have them lying in the left lateral position and get them to curl up into the foetal position. This is where it becomes tricky if the patient is of the larger size. Forward flexion of their lumbar spine opens the intervertebral spaces and allows a path for the needle to pass through. If this is not open then an LP will be impossible. Make sure that their back is just on the edge of the couch and that they are at an adequate height so that you don't have to strain 'upwards' or 'downwards' as you perform the procedure.

Identify the L4/L5 surface landmark by palpating the iliac crests (see the following textbox). Draw an imaginary line between the iliac crests and remember that where this bisects the vertebral body will pass through L4 or

L4/L5. Palpate the vertebral space that you are going to aim for and **mark** with a pen, making sure that you're exactly in the **midline**. Remember that it may palpate easily now but after a bleb of 'local' has been infiltrated the soft tissue anatomy will become distorted making your life much more difficult!

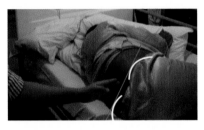

The patient appropriately positioned and the landmarks identified

Wash your hands and **don your sterile gloves**. Using your alcohol cleaning swab or other skin prep liberally **clean the puncture site** and surrounding area. You can then tuck your sterile drape underneath the patient which gives you 'extra' room to work with. If you wish you can take a sterile sheet, cut a hole in the middle and position this over the puncture site, thus creating a **sterile field**.

Now get ready to **inject that local**. Re-check the dose, the expiry date and any allergies. Using a blue (23G) needle, raise a bleb at the surface and give it time to work. Then infiltrate the deeper tissues, focusing on a tract that will pass between the vertebral bodies. The direction you should be aiming for is

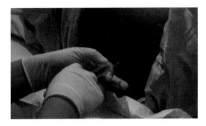

The local anaesthetic infiltrated in the direction the lumbar puncture needle will go

Spinal needles

These come in different sizes and generally you choose them based on patient size and previous attempts! The black is the 'regular size' and is 22G. There are many other colours and sizes, but common ones to be aware of are the yellow 20G (bigger than the black) and the pink 18G (bigger still). The size you choose will also depend on whether this is a therapeutic or diagnostic tap, clearly for a therapeutic tap you will need a bigger needle!

The needle has a bevel and has a 'stylette' running through it which occludes the lumen, mainly to stop bits of fat from blocking the needle. This is removed before obtaining a sample.

You may encounter 'atraumatic' needles at your trust. These can reduce the incidence of Post Dural Puncture Headache. The general consensus seems to be that they reduce the amount of CSF leak from dural puncture post-procedure, and as such reduce the resulting headache. The end of an atraumatic needle is not fashioned as a blade and rather it comes to a point. To decrease the chance of CSF leak further, some clinicians advocate always replacing the stylette before removing the needle as this too may reduce the chance of CSF leak.

towards the umbilicus. Switch to a green (21G) needle and infiltrate deeper still. Make sure always to aspirate as you do so, but don't be too worried-the meninges are deep structures and even with a 'green' you shouldn't be anywhere near them.

Now you are ready to go for the procedure! Take your spinal needle and ensure that the small notch on the plastic part of the stylette is pointing upwards. **Insert the needle** into the skin where you have made a mark and advance it – **aiming towards the umbilicus** always keeping it completely horizontal. You may hit a spinous process which is OK, withdraw and angulate it more cranially or caudally depending on which seems more likely to succeed.

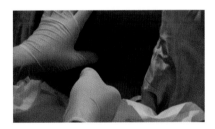

The lumbar puncture needle being inserted

This part really requires practice, but as you pass through the ligamentum flavum you will **feel some resistance**. You're almost there. **Advance the needle** a fraction further and you will feel the resistance give, this is your cue you're in the subarachnoid space. **Withdraw the stylette** and with luck you should have some **CSF dribbling out** of the end of your needle. It often takes quite a few attempts to get CSF, especially when you're starting off but don't be put off-patience usually works!

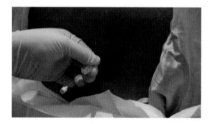

The stylette being withdrawn and a drop of clear CSF appears at the end

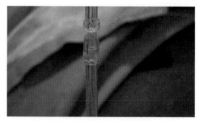

The meniscus of the CSF is seen in the manometer, note the level

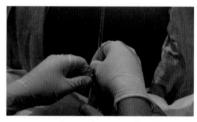

The three-way tap is opened to allow some CSF to drip out into the specimen bottles

At this point ask your assistant to pass you the manometer which you have remembered to preassemble, paying attention to loosen the three-way tap which can be stiff at first. **Attach the manometer** to the spinal needle and you will see the CSF rise within the tube. This 'pressure-meter' simply measures the CSF pressure required to raise a column of fluid-and as such it is measured in cm of water (we assume that CSF has the same density as water). A normal **'opening' pressure** is about 20 cm of water. You will see the meniscus of CSF slowly oscillate with respiration as it reaches equilibrium. Keep a mental note of this and ask your assistant to pass you the first specimen bottle. **Hold the specimen bottle underneath the needle** and empty a few mls of the fluid into it by turning the tap. **Repeat** this with

bottles 2, then 3, then the grey glucose bottle and any other special samples you may have to take.

If you're performing a therapeutic tap you will need to remove more fluid as you're aiming to reduce the CSF pressure. A general rule is to remove enough fluid until the closing pressure is within normal range. The amount will vary. Always measure the closing pressure and document it.

At this point you're done! Carefully **remove the manometer**. **Reinsert the stylette** into the spinal needle before removing it (this has been shown to reduce PDPH) and **apply pressure** with some gauze. **Place a small dressing** over the puncture site.

To finish, make sure that you **label** and send your samples correctly. **Complete your request form** and send it off to the lab. It's vital to also send a **venous glucose** in order to compare it with the CSF glucose (see the following textbox), the CSF and serum samples are called, a **paired sample**. It's good practice to **telephone the lab** and warn them that a paired sample is coming up, particularly out-of-hours as the technician may have to come in to the hospital to take a look at it. Some people always like taking an extra sample to be saved in the fridge in case you wish to request extra tests later, as this saves having to repeat the procedure.

Dispose of your sharps and **document** your procedure in the notes! Make particular note of the CSF appearance: Thick, turbid CSF is not a good sign, nor is blood stained CSF in an atraumatic tap. Also note the opening (and closing if a therapeutic tap) pressure, what tests were sent, whether the procedure was atraumatic or not and a clear plan to follow to action the results. Offer the patient some **postprocedure advice**. The patient may lie down for an hour to give some rest after the procedure but this has not been shown to prevent Post Dural Puncture Headache. On the other hand 'atraumatic' needles have been shown to reduce the risk of such headaches.

Common CSF tests

- Cell count: an automated cell counter or a microbiology technician examines the fluid under the microscope and counts the number of red and white cells per 'field'- normal CSF is sterile and so we would expect less than 5 white cells and less than 10 red cells
- Glucose: this is compared to the serum glucose level and so a **paired** blood sample must always be sent. The general principle is that bacteria 'eat' lots of glucose and so we would expect a relatively low CSF reading whereas a virus would eat less. Hence bacterial meningitis typically has a CSF/Serum glucose of (<1/3). Low glucose readings are also seen in TB and CSF lymphoma.
- Microscopy, culture and sensitivity
- Protein: a high protein level might support GBS for instance
- pH
- Xanthochromia to look for SAH. Make sure to protect your sample from light before sending it to the lab.

- Assembles manometer correctly
- Inserts spinal needle bevel up at correct angle
- Removes stylet
- Obtains CSF
- Attaches manometer, and notes opening pressure
- Takes CSF samples
- Removes spinal needle
- Applies dressing
- Disposes of sharps
- Labels sample bottles
- Advises patient to rest
- Washes hands
- Thanks patient
- Disposes of sharps and waste
- Documents procedure
- Provides postprocedure advice

27 Nasogastric Tube

Video Time | **2 mins 31 s**

Overview

Nasogastric tubes, like any other tube that enters a bodily orifice, can have one of two main purposes. It can be there to put stuff in, or take stuff out. So, NG tubes can be used for **infusing** substances, which for instance could be nutrition, fluids or radiological contrast, or they can be used to **drain** a stomach that requires decompression, usually because of a bowel obstruction. The former require a **fine bore tube** and the latter, a **wide bore tube**.

Although it can often be a straightforward procedure, insertion can sometimes be difficult. The patient may be anxious and this coupled with the patient gagging on the tube can make the whole procedure somewhat tricky and stressful for you and the patient. Talk through the procedure with your patient, look confident and reassure your patient. Gaining their trust and cooperation is key.

It's important to remember that NG tube placement can be potentially dangerous and the indications for tube placement must first be carefully considered. If there is no real clinical need then they should not be used. In addition, try not to request them late in the afternoon or out of hours if possible. Incorrect placement and feeding are 'never-events' and patients have died from this.

Procedure

Make sure you have the **correct patient**, for the **correct procedure**. Check for any **allergies**, and that you have confirmed the **indication;** excluded any **contraindications; explained** the procedure and taken **consent**. Now **wash your hands**!

Assemble all of your equipment on a trolley away from the patient. You will need everything in the equipment textbox.

How to Perform Clinical Procedures, First Edition. Matthew Stephenson, Joshua Shur and John Black.
© 2013 John Wiley & Sons, Ltd. Published 2013 by John Wiley & Sons, Ltd.

Indications	Contraindications	Complications

• Drainage:
  ○ Bowel obstruction
  ○ Paralytic ileus
  ○ Prophylactic
    (eg trauma)
• Feeding:
  ○ Nutrition
  ○ Fluids
  ○ Radiological contrast
	• Base of skull fracture
	• Severe coagulopathy
	• Anatomical deformities
	• Oesophagectomy/
	  gastrectomy
	• Oesophageal varices
		• Epistaxis
		• Mucosal ulceration
		  (with prolonged use)
		• Inappropriate placement
		• Aspiration
		• Infection (sinusitis with
		  prolonged use)

Equipment you need (on a sterile tray/trolley)

- Nasogastric tube (fine bore for feeding, wide bore for drainage)
- Drainage bag
- Lubricating gel
- A 50 ml syringe
- Non-sterile gloves
- Gown
- Cup of water
- Drinking straw
- Adhesive tape
- A vomit bowel
- NPSA accredited pH measuring strip
- Optional – measuring tape

Put on your apron, this procedure is not sterile, but is a **clean** procedure.

It's important to have the patient **positioned correctly**, sat upright with the neck well supported pretty much neutral. A common misconception is that the nasal passage arches upwards and posteriorly. In reality, the nasopharynx falls away inferiorly gradually almost immediately at the point where the tube enters the nose. Check first for any **septal deviation** or obvious nasal obstruction. It can be helpful to ask the patient to gently **blow their nose** prior to the procedure.

Begin by **measuring the length** of tube required to reach the stomach. This is achieved by placing the tip of the tube on the mastoid process, tracing it to the anterior aspect of the mandible (chin), and from the mandible to the xiphisternum. The National Patient Safety Agency (NPSA) recommend a slightly different but equivalent measurement known as the NEX (Nose, Earlobe, Xiphisternum) measurement. This is the tip of the nose to earlobe and then xiphisternum. You need to insert the tube to a minimum of the sum of the two measurements described above, and it may be worth marking the tube at this point. The average distance from nostril to gastrooesophageal junction is 44 cm, and the ideal position within the stomach is about 10 cm below the gastrooesophageal junction. In practice most people will insert the tube approximately

60 cm. You can measure this distance with a measuring tape first, however as NG tubes have length markers it's often easier to just use the tube.

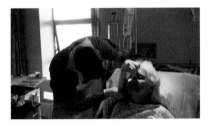

The distance from the nose to the earlobe is being measured

Lubricate the end of the tube but try not to block the holes at the tip of the tube. This will aid passage through the nasal tract. Some clinicians will also squirt some local anaesthetic spray into the nostril beforehand, you can also use lubricating gel that has local anaesthetic in it. Ask the patient to **hold the water** with the drinking straw positioned in their mouth, instructing them to swallow at your request (make sure first to check that they have a safe swallow). Take the lubricated tube in your dominant hand and inflict a slight curve at the tip to imitate the course it is due to take. Warning the patient of an unpleasant sensation at the back of their throat, **advance** the tube postero-inferiorly, asking the patient to begin **swallowing** when they feel the tube at the back of their throat. At this point the passage also becomes a little more difficult (10–15 cm) as you hit the resistance at the back of

the nasopharynx. **Rotating the tube** a little can help as you advance it.

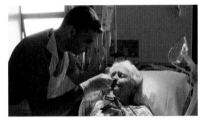

The tube is gently being passed whilst the patient takes sips from their straw

Swallowing encourages the tube down the right lumen (the oesophagus!) by both the action of the pharyngeal constrictors but also by closing the trachea with the epiglottis. **Continue advancing** whilst the patient repeats the swallowing process as often as they comfortably can. If the patient begins to **gag**, this often is a good sign that the tube is travelling in the correct direction. The gagging will stop once the tube goes a little further down the oesohagus. Nevertheless, have a vomit bowl nearby in case. The patient doesn't usually vomit properly but they may retch and spit.

If the patient begins to cough however, you may be intubating the trachea, which is not what you want! **Stop immediately and withdraw** the tube slightly until the coughing subsides. The patient should also be able to talk throughout the procedure, this indicates that there isn't a tube tickling their larynx. If the patient is coughing and unable to swear at you, the tube is going in the wrong direction. You may also notice other signs of respiratory distress. Withdraw, stop the procedure and then try again when the patient has recovered with some more coordinated swallowing and tube advancement.

Occasionally the tube curls up inside the nasopharyngeal space. If you suspect this, **ask the patient to open their mouth** widely – you should be able to see the tube passing down the back of

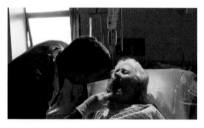

Inspect the oropharynx to ensure the tube has passed through it

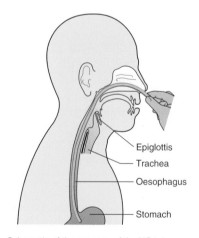

Schematic of the passage of the NG tube

the oropharynx. If you can't see it, it's curled up in the nose, try inserting again in the other nostril. Occasionally you need to **try the other nostril** if there is also resistance to passage through the nasal cavity early on, for instance if the patient has a deviated nasal septum.

Hold the tube in position whilst you fashion some adhesive tape around the NG tube and **anchor it down** to the nasal bridge. Then curve it up over the cheek and over the top of the ipsilateral ear, and tape it in place. Remember there's nothing else to hold that tube in than your tape, there is no balloon for instance as with a urinary catheter, neither you nor the patient will want to go through the whole process again so anchor it well.

If the intra abdominal pressure is high enough and the stomach is filled, you may be greeted by an unwavering flow of bilious stained gastric contents: the importance of wearing gloves and apron, and having a vomit bowel ready! If there's a lot draining, try and **drain** as much as possible into vomit bowls (a syringe can also be used to quickly drain fluid) before attaching the drainage bag which will otherwise just quickly fill up and you'll be doing nothing to relieve the obstruction.

You may not be so lucky to visualise gastric contents coming up the tube, in which case you can **attempt to aspirate** with the 50 ml syringe. You should be able to aspirate a little fluid and air, if not, check the markers on the tube to see if you've advanced as much as you

Epiglottis
Trachea
Oesophagus
Stomach

should. **Try advancing** the tube further into the stomach. Ultimately, if the patient has been vomiting, you may be unable to elicit any aspirate.

There are a few ways of **confirming the position** of the NG tube, that is, ensuring that it isn't coiled up in the oesophagus, or rarely, somehow got into the respiratory tract.

If the tube is placed in the correct location, an aspirate should be acidic. If a successful aspirate has been obtained, the **pH** can be tested using **NPSA compliant pH testing strips**. The pH MUST be 5.5 or less for feeding to confirm placement in the stomach. Carefully expel a minimum of 0.5 ml from the syringe onto a strip. If the fluid has originated from the stomach the pH will be 5.5 or less.

The NPSA also suggest lying the patient on their left side and waiting 20–30 minutes to encourage an aspirate. **Do not flush the tube with water** before confirming placement – the tube may not be in the correct position. A recent NPSA alert (March 2012) also noted that flushing a lubricated tube can result in a mixture with a pH of <5.5. If you were to then aspirate to confirm placement this could potentially erroneously suggest that you were in the stomach.

Ultimately, the **gold standard** is to visualise the radiolucent tube tip by means of a **chest x-ray**. The NPSA flow chart clearly states to proceed to x-ray if gastric aspirate is not obtained or pH testing is not within 1–5.5. If the tube

has been located correctly, the tip should be visible on the chest x-ray, lying below the diaphragm and clear of the lung fields. **Under no circumstances should any fluid or feed be administered via the tube until you have absolute evidence of its placement with aspirate of pH of 5.5 or less or radiological evidence**. This should be documented clearly in the notes and communicated with all clinical staff involved in the patient's care. Most importantly, **check your trust's guidelines** and make sure you are adhering to them.

Finally, **disconnect the syringe** from the tube, **connect the drainage bag** and dispose of your clinical waste. **Wash your hands** and **document** the procedure clearly in the clinical notes. Include the length of tube introduced, the results of any aspiration or chest x-ray and the indication for placing the NG tube. Have a clear plan for the tube including who is responsible for checking that placement is confirmed.

Spigoting the NG tube

Later, once the obstruction has been decompressed, or paralytic ileus begins to resolve for instance, you may wish to **spigot the tube**, rendering it functionless. Spigoting the tube just means putting a cap (spigot) on the end. This enables the tube to be left in, and the option of further decompression if required. Clinically, if the obstruction appears to be resolving, the tube can be removed after 24 hours. Spigoting the tube and assessing in this way before withdrawal may minimise the chances of having to reinsert it.

Decision tree for nasogastric tube placement checks in ADULTS

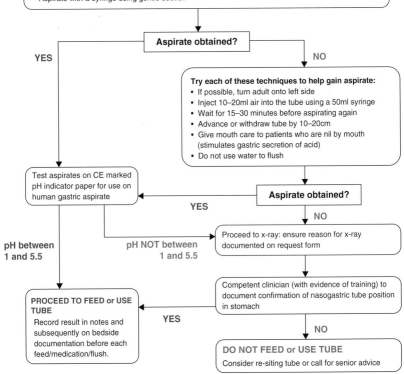

- Estimate NEX measurment (Place exit port of tube at tip of nose. Extend tube to earlobe, and then to xiphisternum)
- Insert fully radio-opaque nasogastric tube for feeding (follow manufacturer's instructions for insertion)
- Confirm and document secured NEX measurment
- Aspirate with a syringe using gentle suction

Aspirate obtained?

YES   NO

Try each of these techniques to help gain aspirate:
- If possible, turn adult onto left side
- Inject 10–20ml air into the tube using a 50ml syringe
- Wait for 15–30 minutes before aspirating again
- Advance or withdraw tube by 10–20cm
- Give mouth care to patients who are nil by mouth (stimulates gastric secretion of acid)
- Do not use water to flush

Test aspirates on CE marked pH indicator paper for use on human gastric aspirate

Aspirate obtained?

YES   NO

Proceed to x-ray: ensure reason for x-ray documented on request form

pH between 1 and 5.5   pH NOT between 1 and 5.5

Competent clinician (with evidence of training) to document confirmation of nasogastric tube position in stomach

PROCEED TO FEED or USE TUBE
Record result in notes and subsequently on bedside documentation before each feed/medication/flush.

YES   NO

DO NOT FEED or USE TUBE
Consider re-siting tube or call for senior advice

A pH of between 1 and 5.5 is reliable confirmation that the tube is not in the lung, however it does not confirm gastric placement as there is a small chance the tube tip may sit in the oesophagus where it carries a higher risk of aspiration. If this is any concern, the patient should proceed to x-ray in order to confirm tube position.

Where pH readings fall between 5 and 6 it is recommended that a second competent person checks the reading or retests.

Rapid Response Report

NPSA/2012/RRR001

From reporting to learning   22 March 2012

Harm from flushing of nasogastric tubes before confirmation of placement

Issue

Misplaced nasogastric tubes leading to death or severe harm are 'never events.' The Patient Safety Alert *Reducing the harm caused by misplaced nasogastric feeding tubes in adults, children and infants* was issued by the NPSA on 10 March 2011 with an action complete date of 12 September 2011. Alongside other actions, this Alert requires all organisations to ensure that *"Nasogastric tubes are not flushed, nor any liquid/feed introduced through the tube following initial placement, until the tube tip is confirmed by pH testing or x-ray to be in the stomach."* This advice is repeated in the National Nurses Nutrition Group *Good Practice Guideline: Safe Insertion of Nasogastric Feeding Tubes in Adults.*

The advice not to flush until after gastric placement is confirmed is important because:
- any flush could cause an aspiration pneumonia if the tube is misplaced in the lungs;
- pH testing for gastric placement relies on collecting aspirate via the tube; anything introduced down the tube will contaminate this aspirate, potentially leading to false positive pH readings.

Evidence of harm

The NPSA is aware of two patient deaths since 10 March 2011 where staff had flushed nasogastric tubes with water before initial placement had been confirmed. Staff then aspirated back the water they had flushed into the tube, including the lubricant within the tube that this water had activated. Because this mix of water and lubricant gave a pH reading below 5.5, they assumed that the nasogastric tube was correctly placed and went on to give medications and/or feed, although the tube was actually in the patient's lung. We are also aware of a similar incident which did not lead to harm to a patient.

The three organisations where the incidents occurred were aware of the NPSA Alert, but there appeared to be a widespread belief amongst their frontline staff that the 'never flush' rule did not apply where nasogastric tubes had a water-activated lubricant. This belief is incorrect, and the manufacturer's written guidance, enclosed with each new nasogastric tube, clearly states that gastric placement must be confirmed BEFORE the tube is flushed. The lubricant is not needed for placement, only to aid removal of the guidewire/ stylet from the tube **after gastric placement has been confirmed**.

FOR IMMEDIATE ACTION by all organisations in the NHS and independent sector where nasogastric feeding tubes are placed and used for feeding patients. The deadline for action complete is 21 September 2012.

1. Assign a named clinical lead to coordinate implementation of the actions in this Rapid Response Report (RRR) with any actions outstanding from the earlier Alert
2. Remind all staff responsible for checking initial placement of nasogastric tubes (including staff who support parents/carers who check initial placement of nasogastric tubes):
    a. NOTHING should be introduced down the tube before gastric placement has been confirmed;
    b. DO NOT FLUSH the tube before gastric placement has been confirmed;
    c. Internal guidewires/ stylets should NOT be lubricated before gastric placement has been confirmed.
3. This reminder should be given through:
    a. Distributing this RRR to all relevant staff;
    b. Providing warning notices and/ or overwraps with warning labels on all current and future stock of nasogastric tubes, until these are provided as standard by manufacturers;
    c. Reviewing and, if necessary, amending all local policy, protocol and training materials.

The NPSA has alerted device manufacturers of this risk and will promote the need for safer design and labelling. Any concerns related to manufacturers' instructions for use or labelling should be reported to the Medicines and Healthcare products Regulatory Agency.

NHS Evidence
accredited provider
NHS Evidence - provided by NICE
www.evidence.nhs.uk

Further information: This RRR should be read in conjunction with the previous Alert *Reducing the harm caused by misplaced nasogastric feeding tubes in adults, children and infants.* This remains in force and should be referred to for all other issues, including repeat placement checks after initial gastric placement has been confirmed. For further queries contact rrr@npsa.nhs.uk, Telephone 020 7927 9500.

28 Nebuliser

Video Time | 1 min 41 s

Overview

Nebulisers have been used in modern clinical practice since the 19th century. From the latin for *mist*, they essentially vaporise a drug and deliver it to its therapeutic target deep within the lungs. Nebulisers are **exceedingly common** literally hundreds or thousands of nebules per day are likely to be consumed in a large teaching hospital. In the community, home nebulisers are used in the households of many chronic airways disease patients.

Why is it important that you know how to use one? Simply because they are **common** and **important** in the treatment (and diagnosis) of respiratory disease: particularly **asthma** and **COPD**. *And* setting one up will make you a hit with your nursing colleagues. More importantly, if your patient is experiencing severe breathlessness due to wheeze – are you going to stand there twiddling your thumbs whilst you wait for the nurse? Hope not.

Before understanding the correct usage of a nebuliser it's important first to understand the basic mechanism of how a nebuliser works. It's worth noting that there are countless varieties of nebuliser but this is the basic principle:

- The nebuliser 'box' compresses the feeding gas (either air or oxygen) to increase its pressure. If you're using oxygen you will need to connect the box to the wall oxygen.
- The compressed gas passes through a small hole (known as a Venturi) at which point its pressure drops and it expands. This creates a negative pressure around the surrounding nebule fluid.
- During gas expansion the liquid in the surrounding chamber is vapourised and carried out of the reservoir as the patient takes a breath.

How to Perform Clinical Procedures, First Edition. Matthew Stephenson, Joshua Shur and John Black.
© 2013 John Wiley & Sons, Ltd. Published 2013 by John Wiley & Sons, Ltd.

- Larger fluid droplets recondense (on something called a baffle) to be eventually revapourised however the smaller droplets are carried into the lungs on inspiration. This raises some important points:
- Whatever gas you feed the nebuliser your patient will eventually breath in. This is important in COPD patients.
- The flow rate of gas needs to be controlled. If it's too high it will be uncomfortable for the patient.
- The higher the flow rate the smaller the vapourised gas – and an effective particle size of about 1–5 microns needs to be reached. In addition, the higher the flow rate the quicker the liquid will be vapourised!

So what are nebulisers actually used for? By far the most common reasons that you would prescribe a nebuliser is for the treatment of the common obstructive respiratory diseases: asthma and COPD with a **bronchodilator** – normally a beta-agonist (e.g. *salbumatol*) or anti-muscarinic (e.g. *ipratropium*). Many will also have prescribed or come across simple **saline** nebulisers as a mucolytic, for instance in patients with lots of secretions, to help break these up.

Bronchodilator therapy is commonly used in primary care for patients requiring nebulisers, and in secondary care for both **chronic airways disease management**, or in the **acute management** of an exacerbation of one of these diseases.

The first common indication for nebulising a drug is typically when a patient is **too ill** to use any other inhaled therapy (such as acute severe asthma). In this case a patient will simply be too unwell to comply with other therapies.

The second case is when an extremely **high dose** of medication is required – such that it can only be practically delivered by nebuliser. This might be the case when a patient is required to use their conventional inhaler far in excess of what is normal practice.

It can be seen that most severely unwell patients requiring bronchodilator therapy will fit into both of the above indications.

A further indication for nebuliser therapy is when a drug **requires nebulisation** as a route (there being no alternative). As a junior doctor however this is something less commonly encountered, the most common drugs that fall into this category are used in cystic fibrosis (for example some nebulised antibiotics or rhDNase in sputum retention).

For those that are interested, many drugs can be delivered by nebuliser including steroids, antibiotics, local anaesthetics etc. In addition nebulisers can be used as a diagnostic tool. In the realms of nuclear medicine, radioactive particles are nebulised and inhaled to image a patient's ventilation. This is one part of the V/Q or ventilation/perfusion scan.

As you know nebuliser therapy needs to be prescribed, like any other drug. The key things you need to remember here is the **drug dose**, **gas you are driving** it with and **frequency**.

With respect to the dose, by far the most common drugs you will prescribe will be **salbutamol** (or another short acting beta-agonist) and **ipratropium** (or another anti-cholinergic). The doses for these are usually 2.5–5 mg for salbutamol and 500 micrograms for ipatropium – remember these two – you will use them a lot!

With respect to the gas the main thing to remember with **asthma**: always drive the nebuliser with **oxygen**. With **COPD**, drive the nebuliser with **air** and use supervised oxygen therapy (the risk of course being the rare dampening of a patient's hypoxic respiratory drive).

In summary: Asthma = Oxygen, COPD = Air.

What about frequency? Well as part of maintenance therapy both drugs are traditionally given a maximum of **four times daily**. In the acute setting, however, you will probably be aware that Salbutamol can be given '**back to back**' (i.e. continuously). However, be aware that your patient will most likely develop a tremor and tachycardia!

Indications	Contraindications	Complications
• Unwell patient unable to comply with conventional inhalers. • When large amounts of drug is required to be delivered by inhalation. • When nebulisation is only suitable administration route.	• Allergy to the nebulised drug	• Allergic reaction • Drug specific side effects

Procedure

Make sure you have the **correct patient**, for this procedure. Check for any **allergies**, and that you have confirmed the **indication;** excluded any **contraindications;** explained the procedure and taken **consent**. Now **wash your hands**!

Assemble all of your equipment on a trolley. You will need everything in the equipment textbox.

Equipment you need (on a sterile tray/trolley)

- Nebuliser box (air compressor)
- Appropriate face mask
- Nebule
- Nebuliser chamber

Connect the nebuliser chamber to the nebuliser box using the plastic tubing.

There are different chambers available but in most cases you will need to unscrew it and **fill it with the nebule** (e.g. salbutamol). Always remember to check the drug before filling the chamber. Make sure that you keep the chamber held **vertically** as otherwise the liquid will spill out.

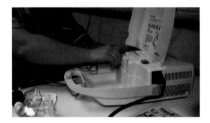

The tubing is connected to the machine which is plugged in and switched on

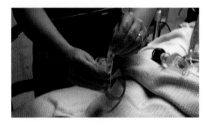

Fill the nebuliser chamber with the drug

Next, **connect an appropriate mouthpiece** or facemask to the nebuliser cup. Most commonly this will be a standard facemask. In theory there are considerations that need to be taken into account with this respect-for example a mouthpiece is more desirable when using a nebulised steroid to avoid unnecessary steroid deposition around the mouth, or even in the eyes.

Turn the nebuliser on and ensure it's working correctly. If you're driving the nebuliser with oxygen then **connect it to the wall oxygen**. Ensure that your patient is **sat upright** (to improve access of the nebulised drug to the lung bases too) and place the mask comfortably over their face. The patient should be asked to **breath as normal** and **avoid talking** too much.

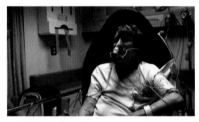

The nebuliser attached to the mask, which is on the patient

During the procedure ask the patient to **tap on the chamber** once in a while to prevent condensation.

As for some of the reasons mentioned before, delivery time will vary however a typical time is around **5–10 minutes**. A clue that you have reached the end is when the nebuliser starts 'sputtering'. This is a sign that there is not enough liquid left to properly vapourise. **Turn off the machine** and **remove the facemask**. You will notice that there will be some liquid left in the cup at the end-and you may be surprised how much this is compared to what you put in! Nebuliser design thus tries to minimise this 'residual' so as to maximise the amount of drug delivered to the patient. If the patient was requiring oxygen before the nebuliser, remember to re-attach it and not put them back just on room air!

It's unlikely that you will have to clean or maintain the nebuliser machine your-self, and as they vary so much in design it's best to refer to the manufacturers guidelines for this. However, make sure that you have **signed the prescription chart** to say that you've given the drug.

OSCE checklist

- Checks and assembles nebuliser airbox
- Unscrews nebuliser mask
- Checks drug dose, name and expiry date
- Squirts drug into nebuliser vault
- Reassembles nebuliser
- Secures mask on patient comfortably
- Turns on nebuliser
- Removes mask once nebuliser is finished
- Washes hands
- Thanks patient

29 Observations

Video Time | 2 mins 9 s

Overview

Observations (often shortened to just 'Obs'), or in North America 'Vital Signs' or 'Vitals' are the most important basic measurable parameters that are used in clinical practice.

Who gets their observations taken? *Everyone*. It forms one of the basic pillars of clinical assessment along with a thorough history and examination. Every patient who attends hospital will at the very least require a full set of initial observations.

Observations are almost always performed in secondary care by nursing staff, and indeed nowadays the trend is towards less trained nursing staff (for example healthcare assistants) to perform this vital function. This is because it's a relatively simple task, and it can free trained nursing staff to perform other jobs.

So then why does a doctor need to know how to take observations? Well there are a number of good reasons:

- In the acutely ill patient you may need to quickly obtain a set of observations – doing this yourself is much easier than waiting for a busy nurse to do it for you. Indeed there may be opportunities simply when the nurses are unavailable and you **need** to do it yourself.
- When interpreting any test result (for example body temperature) it's important to have a basic understanding of the measuring device (i.e. thermometer). This is so you can appreciate the limitations, accuracy, precision and common pitfalls that accompany **any** test.
- In primary care you will often have to perform a quick set of observations during the consultation-if you want to be a GP it's good to get into this habit early.

How to Perform Clinical Procedures, First Edition. Matthew Stephenson, Joshua Shur and John Black.
© 2013 John Wiley & Sons, Ltd. Published 2013 by John Wiley & Sons, Ltd.

In addition, it forces you to get close to your patient and take notice of them. This is one of the main arguments against the decline in trained nurses taking observations. Some nurses complain that they now get less opportunity to interact with their patients and potentially spot any problems early.

When we talk about observations we are referring to five basic clinical parameters:

1 Body temperature

2 Blood pressure

3 Pulse rate

4 Respiratory rate

5 Peripheral oxygen saturations

(Some people include a sixth 'AVPU' (**A**lert, responding to **V**oice, responding to **P**ain, **U**nresponsive) score which is a basic measurement of conscious level – however, we won't be discussing this further).

The scope of this chapter is not to discuss these each in detail (particularly in what situations they may change), rather it will outline how to measure each of these in turn using common equipment, and any particular tips to keep in mind.

For a general acute medical or surgical ward, the minimum that a patient will have their observations taken is four times per day. More unwell patients may have them done at 4-hourly, 2-hourly or more frequent intervals. Indeed patients requiring frequent or continuous monitoring is an indication for level 2 (HDU) or level 3 (ICU) care.

It's important to mention that a snapshot of observations in time is **often not helpful**, what is far better is to observe the **trend** of the observations over a period of time. A good example of this is the development of early warning scoring systems such as **NEWS** (National Early Warning Score). Very briefly-observations are given an individual score depending on their deviation from 'normal'. These are then summated to give a total score for a patient. This score can then be used to trigger specific actions, such as calling a doctor. This is useful as a **screening tool** to escalate care when a patient may be deteriorating. However their use must be taken into context-for some perfectly well people, their 'normal' observations may score highly on an early warning score. These people simply lie to the 'edge of the bell-curve'. What this means in practice is that you will get a lot of calls from nurses if their patient's NEWS score is high-this will trigger you to examine the patient and properly determine how unwell they may be.

It's difficult to over-emphasise the importance of thorough clinical observations and accurate recording in the clinical notes. It's vital to making a proper assessment of a patient, and it's often infuriating when looking at the observations folder if it's incomplete. Try and insist on proper observations and record-keeping, even if this means doing it yourself!

Procedure

Make sure you have the **correct patient**, for the **correct procedure**. Check that you have confirmed the **indication** and that you've excluded any **contraindications** (e.g. checking the blood pressure on an arm with an arteriovenous fistula for dialysis) and taken verbal **consent**. Now **wash your hands**!

Temperature

There are a variety of ways and sites to record body temperature. Traditional sites include oral, axillary, rectal, tympanic, vaginal and over the temporal artery. It's known that the site of measurement can affect the reading-indeed 'internal' measurements such as rectal or vaginal will usually read about 1° of Fahrenheit above other sites.

Historically, the gold standard has been the rectal mercury thermometer. This is partly because the rectal temperature is considered to be an accurate reflection of the **core** temperature, which ultimately we are trying to measure.

Mercury thermometers were replaced with electronic probes and more recently (since the early 1990s) the method of choice has been with a tympanic infra-red thermometer. This is currently the most commonly used method, primarily due to the fact it is quick and simple to use (the 'old' mercury thermometers might take *minutes* whereas a tympanic thermometer can take *seconds*). The tympanic membrane is well perfused, and its proximity to the brain means that it's accepted as a good representation of core temperature. Rather than touch the membrane, the probe measures infrared energy (i.e. heat) radiating from the structure and converts this to a temperature.

Although it's not **the** most accurate of methods, it's preferred for its convenience.

Seeing as the probe measures radiated heat, there are a few things to consider. Firstly excessive wax (we mean lots!) or if the probe is not facing the tympanic membrane may cause an inaccurate result. Fluid behind the eardrum (such as a middle ear effusion) may also interfere with the reading. In addition the probe is usually too large for small children and so is not generally used in children under the age of two.

Indications	Contraindications	Complications
• For measurement of core temperature	• Ear trauma • Recent ear surgery-check with a senior • Young children (under 2 years)	• Ear drum perforation (rare but reported)

Although designs differ, measuring body temperature with a tympanic thermometer is similar between different models.

First **inspect the ear canal** to check for any blood or ear trauma. If you are satisfied it's safe to proceed, remove the thermometer from its stand and have a look at the end of the probe to **check that it's clean**. Push the probe into a **plastic probe cover** until it clicks – this indicates it's in place. Gently **place the probe into the ear canal**, aiming to angle it towards the tympanic membrane. There will be a button on the back of the thermometer to take the reading – **press the button** and bingo, it works in seconds. **Remove the probe**, and **dispose of the cover**. There should be another release button that pops it off.

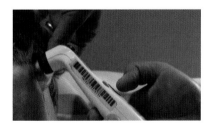

The tympanic membrane temperature probe in position

Finally **record the temperature** in the clinical notes.

If you think the reading may be inaccurate then check that the probe is clean and that you have positioned it correctly.

> ### Equipment you need to measure body temperature
> - Tympanic thermometer
> - Disposable probe cover

Blood pressure

Blood pressure is measured with a sphygmomanometer (Sphygmo – *from the greek for pulse* and manometer – *pressure measuring device*), often shortened to 'sphyg' for convenience.

Sphygs are usually divided into **manual** and **electronic** devices. Electronic sphygs are used routinely in clinical practice (mainly for their convenience); however, if they are unable to record a pressure then a manual device is often used as a second line.

Manual sphygs consist of an inflatable pressure cuff and require you to **auscultate** just distal to the cuff. As we remember the cuff 'squeezes' the artery, disrupting laminar blood flow and resulting in audible turbulence that we are interested in hearing (the eponymous *Korotkoff* sounds). Needless to say the main difference between manual sphygs is the method of pressure measurement (for example with an aneroid (clock-face dial) or column of mercury). A complete description of the technique of manual blood pressure measurement is outside the scope of this book so we will leave you to look this up if you can't remember it.

Rather, as electronic sphygs are so frequently used nowadays we will concentrate on describing their use. **Electronic** sphygs work completely differently. There is no auscultation used, rather the machine detects pulsations in the arterial wall due to turbulent flow through the artery under pressure.

As normal, the cuff is inflated (this time electronically by the machine) to just above the systolic blood pressure. As we remember, at this pressure the artery is completely occluded and there is no arterial blood flow. Again the cuff slowly deflates and as the cuff pressure decreases just below the systolic pressure, the onset of turbulent flow causes increased vibrations within the arterial wall. These vibrations are transmitted through the blood pressure cuff where they are turned into electronic signals which are sent to the machine (for those that are interested, piezoelectric crystals are used which cause a tiny voltage difference across them when they are deformed). This electrical signal continues as the cuff deflates, to the point at which the diastolic blood pressure is reached. At this point laminar blood flow is restored and the vibrations stop (in practice life is never so simple, and in fact the oscillatory signal gradually increases as systole is reached up to the MAP and then gradually decreases to pass diastole – as there will always be a background oscillatory component; however the general principle applies!).

To operate the machine first **expose your patient's upper arm** and **place the cuff** around it. One side will be marked to face the patient's arm and you should ensure that you do so. **Secure the cuff** and **press the inflate button**-hey presto! The cuff can also be placed around the leg if needed.

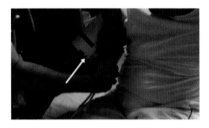

The blood pressure cuff is placed around the upper arm

The advantages of an electronic sphyg is that cuff placement and size is much less of an issue. It is also essentially operator independent. The disadvantages are that certain arrythmias can cause problems and that 'stiff' arteries may also interfere with readings. As a general baseline blood pressure however it's satisfactory. If the machine does have difficulty remember a manual reading can always be taken.

Pulse and oxygen saturations

Pulse rate is nowadays commonly measured electronically during the nursing 'observations' round. Of course, it's easy to take your patients hand and palpate their radial pulse and we would always advocate that approach!

To outline the 'electronic' method, the pulse is inferred from measuring the blood haemoglobin oxygen saturations

Indications	Contraindications	Complications
• For measurement of blood pressure	• Not for neonates or young babies! • Arrythmias (depending on machine) • Trauma to arm • Arteriovenous fistula in arm • Previous ipsilateral axillary node clearance for breast cancer (relative)	• Inaccuracy in certain conditions

with a **pulse oximeter**. Since the saturation varies with arterial pulsation, a waveform is produced. From this, the pulse rate can be calculated.

Modern pulse oximeters work by shining light through tissue that is perfused, such as a finger, toe or earlobe. It turns out that oxyhaemoglobin and deoxyhaemoglobin absorb light differently, and by measuring this difference an estimation of oxygen saturations can be calculated.

The advantages of this method is that it's quick and easy and is suitable for non-invasive continuous monitoring.

Disadvantages are that adequate tissue perfusion is required as such hypoperfusion can give inaccurate readings – essentially it must pick up a pulsatile waveform to work. In addition, a normal oxygen saturation can be misleading. For example an anaemic patient may have a normal or high oxygen saturation. Carbon monoxide poisoning can cause reassuringly high oxygen saturations, despite the fact that tissues are not receiving any oxygen. In addition nail varnishes or lacquers can also interfere so make sure you remove them first!

So how do you use one? Simply **place the oximeter probe** on your patient's finger or toe and **turn the machine on**! For neonates there are smaller probes which can be stuck around a finger. The machine will need to register 4 or 5 pulsations at first to obtain a reading so be patient. It will then return the pulse rate.

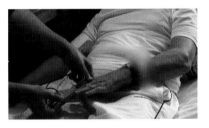

The pulse oximeter placed on the finger

Respiratory rate

Respiratory rate is one of the more sensitive observations recorded. Therefore it's important to measure it accurately and act on any adverse signs. Whilst this can be measured electronically, it's conventionally measured manually. Observe the patient's chest for rise and fall; if they are wearing a mask, their exhalation will

Indications	Contraindications	Complications
• For measurement of pulse and oxygen saturations.	• Caution should be used in shocked patients who are hypoperfused, in anaemia, carbon monoxide poisoning or in cold or tremulous digits.	• Prolonged use may cause abrasion or blistering of the finger-tips (rare).

normally 'fog' it. Where breathing is shallow, a hand can be placed on the anterior chest wall to palpate for expansion if there is any ambiguity.

Once you're confident you have established the patient's respiratory rhythm, **begin counting** the number of respirations in 1 minute with the aid of a time keeping device. It's acceptable to count the number of respirations in 30 seconds and multiply up by two if you are short on time. Simultaneously listen for any harsh respiratory noises or signs of respiratory distress which may need addressing. Ensure the respiratory rate gets recorded on the observations chart. Observe for any dramatic shifts to the trend and act on them appropriately.

OSCE checklist

- Places blood pressure cuff correctly
- Attaches cuff to machine
- Places pulse oximeter correctly
- Switches on observation machine
- Records BP, pulse and Sats correctly
- Records temperature correctly
- Counts respiration rate correctly
- Washes hands
- Thanks patient

30 Peak Flow Rate

Video Time | 1 min 34 s

Overview

Measuring peak flow (strictly peak expiratory flowrate) is a simple, non-invasive measure of respiratory function. It's most often performed by your nursing colleagues; however, it's important that as a junior doctor you are competent at performing it.

This is for a number of reasons:

- It is one of your **core procedures** as a foundation doctor for which you are required to prove competence.
- It's used both in **diagnosis** and **monitoring** of **asthma** (and to a lesser degree **COPD)**.
- These diseases are important in **both primary and secondary care**, so wherever you end up working you may need to perform this test and interpret the results.

Peak flow is a measure of **maximum air flow rate** that can be produced in a forced expiration. Flow is generally measured in the units of volume/time and as such peak flow is measured in litres per minute (L/min). In obstructive airways disease (for example asthma or COPD) the airway cross-sectional area is reduced and (courtesy of Jean Louis Marie Poiseuille we know that non-turbulent flow is proportional to the radius to the fourth power so air flow will also be reduced. So we can infer the degree of airway obstruction from the degree of peak flow.

The meter itself is 'prescribable' and you will no doubt encounter the 'Wright' or 'mini-wright' peak flow meter. Things, however, are complicated slightly by the fact that there have been attempts over the years to standardise peak flow meters scales. The net result is that there are different colours of the standard meter for the different flow scales. The one you will almost certainly use will be the European standard meter which

How to Perform Clinical Procedures, First Edition. Matthew Stephenson, Joshua Shur and John Black.
© 2013 John Wiley & Sons, Ltd. Published 2013 by John Wiley & Sons, Ltd.

will have blue text on a yellow background. If you are unsure check the manufacturer's leaflet and it should note that it's compliant with the EU 13826 standard.

> For those that are interested, the gentleman who invented the peak flow meter was Dr Wright, a British engineer back in the Fifties. Since then the meter has undergone a series of revisions and updates, including smaller versions 'the mini-wright' and low-flow versions. These meters were measured in the 'Wright' scale; however, since 2004 we have adopted a standardised EU scale basically to improve meter accuracy. Why is any of this relevant? Well 1 Wright does not equal exactly 1 EU. If you have an older patient who switched in 2004 to the new meter then it may seem that their peak flow has suddenly dropped; however, it's simply due to a change of scale. For any patient who started using their meter since 2004 however this is unlikely to be relevant any more.

So when will you perform peak flow? Well the BTS recommend using it:

1 As an aid to the **diagnosis of asthma** in adults. The peak flow before and after bronchodilator therapy is particularly useful as a guide for airway reversibility.

2 The **percentage predicted** peak flow is also used to **categorise** acute severe asthma and guide how aggressive your initial treatment should be.

3 In the community, peak flow can also be used to **monitor** the condition and can be recorded in a diary – diurnal variation is strongly suggestive of asthma.

With respect to COPD, the BTS also recommend peak flow as an additional investigation to **differentiate** COPD from asthma-particularly with a peak flow **diary** looking for any evidence of diurnal variation.

It's worth mentioning that in young children, peak flow readings can be unreliable as a degree of cooperation is needed with the 'instructor' – for that reason their readings should be taken with a 'pinch of salt'.

Indications	Contraindications	Complications
• Diagnosis and management of asthma and COPD	• None	• Mild initial breathlessness

Equipment you need

- Peak flow meter
- Nomogram
- Disposable mouthpiece

Procedure

Make sure you have the **correct patient**, for the **correct procedure**. When instructing your patient you must ensure that they are **holding the meter**

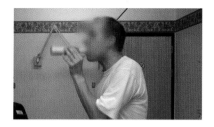
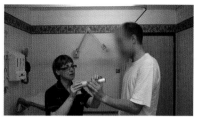

Ask the patient to stand up and exhale as quickly and forcefully as possible

Check the reading on the meter

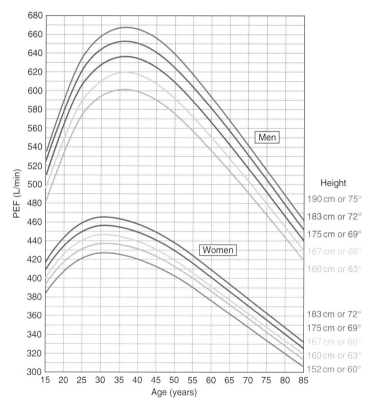

Nomogram of the peak flow rates per age, sex and height
(*Source*: A.J. Nunn and I. Gregg (1989) *Br. Med. J.* **298**: 1068–70. Reproduced with permission of BMJ Publishing)

correctly. Essentially they can hold it any way they please as long as they aren't stopping the peak-flow 'pointer' from sliding along the meter. This point is very important.

Carefully **explain** that you want the patient to **exhale as quickly and forcefully** as they can. Sometimes demonstrating this can help. Remind them to keep a **good seal** around the mouthpiece.

Insert a disposable mouthpiece, ask them to **stand** or sit up straight, take a deep breath in, place the meter in their mouth and then **exhale as forcefully** as possible. Note the reading and then **repeat it two further times** after resetting the meter, which is simply done by sliding the pointer back to zero. You're looking for the **best reading of the three**. Dispose of the mouthpiece and **clean** the meter. This can be done with warm soapy water and left to air dry.

Have a look at the patient's best reading and their corresponding 'normal' value. The normal value is calculated from the **nomogram** based on the patient's sex, height and age.

For example: If you're using an EU scale 'mini-wright' and your 175 cm tall, 50-year-old male patient had a peak flow of about 310 L/min then looking at the nomogram you will see that their predicted is 620 L/min (so they have registered 50% of predicted).

OSCE checklist
- Explains technique to patient
- Attaches mouth piece and sets counter to zero
- Asks patient to stand
- Performs three readings
- Uses nomogram to calculate normal PEF for age, sex and height
- Washes hands
- Thanks patient

31 Peripheral Venous Cannulation

Video Time | 3 mins 33 s

Overview

Siting a cannula (aka the venflon, aka a drip) is probably *the* most important skill to learn after taking blood. Why is it so important? Simply because we do so many of them and that so much of medicine requires ready access to the circulation.

'Gaining access' is important for many reasons: A patient may be dry, necessitating intravenous rehydration. They may require medication to be administered through a drip. They may even require blood to be given through a drip. In general *any* sick patient will require a cannula and it's part of the 'sick patient package' that will be requested (along with bloods, chest x-ray, catheter, BM, ECG +/– a few others depending on the situation).

As a junior doctor you will be asked to do hundreds if not thousands of them. Indeed it is (usually!) not a difficult procedure and many nurses are now trained to cannulate. Keep a mental note of these nurses as they can usually help you out in tricky situations! In addition most site practitioners can cannulate and if you are having trouble give them a call. However, as mentioned in the venepuncture chapter – don't miss out on the opportunity to practise cannulating just because there are so many other people who are able to do it. Intravenous cannulation is an absolutely basic prerequisite for being a useful junior doctor. You'll look like a numpty at the inevitable cardiac arrest call when you're stumbling around trying to get a line in because you haven't had the practice. If there's a cannula to be put in and you're free – do it yourself! The learning curve for doing the most difficult cannulae requires experience in the order of hundreds.

Before we start going through the procedure it's probably worth discussing the equipment in more detail. As you are probably aware, a cannula is a small plastic tube

How to Perform Clinical Procedures, First Edition. Matthew Stephenson, Joshua Shur and John Black.
© 2013 John Wiley & Sons, Ltd. Published 2013 by John Wiley & Sons, Ltd.

Indications	Contraindications	Complications
• For administration of intravenous products: Fluid, medications, blood etc. Can be performed preemptively if a patient is likely to deteriorate.	Essentially the same for venepuncture: • Mastectomy – patients who have had mastectomy +/– an axillary clearance • Phlebitis (or any other localised infection) • AV fistula • Distal to site of previous cannula (caution) • Paralysed limb (caution)	• Bleeding/haematoma/bruising • Phlebitis – can be serious. Nowadays cannula care sheets and regular nursing observation are used to pick this up early. • Extravasation or 'tissuing'. This is when cannula contents start entering the surrounding tissue rather than vein. Commonly occurs in people with *poor* veins or after prolonged use of a cannula • Damage to surrounding structures, e.g. artery, nerve. • Cannula embolism: This is very rare but a theoretical complication if a part of the cannula gets broken off and embolises into the vein.

that sits in the vein. It's common sense to say that there are some situations in which a big tube will be needed and some in which a smaller tube will be required – the bigger the tube the quicker 'stuff' can be put into the vein.

For example, a patient is admitted to resus with a massive upper GI bleed. Do you want a small piddly cannula or a massive drainpipe? The answer is **two** massive drainpipes, such as grey (16G) or even brown (14G), one in each antecubital fossa. What about the elderly patient with tiny veins who needs a bit of IV antibiotics now and again? We can probably suffice with a pink (20G) or even a blue (22G) cannula. As we (may) be aware, Poiseuille's law states that flow through a tube varies with the radius to the fourth power! (this means if you double the width of the tube the flow rate goes up by 16 times). Cannula 'widths' (or gauges) are coloured to distinguish them. From smallest to largest there is most commonly yellow (24G) blue (22G), pink (20G), green (18G) and grey (16G).

So in essence the main point we are trying to make is: select your cannula wisely, for the situation for which it is required. The principle is to select a cannula that will deliver the required flow rate and cannulate a vein that is large enough to withstand the procedure. The cannula should theoretically 'float' in the vein as good haemodilution of the drug and sufficient flow rate of blood return is important.

Procedure

Make sure you have the **correct patient**, for the **correct procedure**. Check for any **allergies** (unlikely to be an issue in this procedure), and that you have confirmed the **indication;** excluded any **contraindications; explained** the procedure and taken **consent**. Now **wash your hands**!

Assemble all of your equipment on a trolley away from the patient. You will need everything in the equipment textbox.

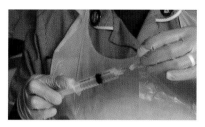

Drawing up the saline flush. In some hospitals this comes prepackaged already drawn up

Equipment you will need (on a clean tray/trolley)

- Intravenous cannula
- Saline flush
- Syringe to draw up flush
- Some sterile gauze
- Sterile swab
- A plastic bung/cap or needle free connector and extension set
- Adhesive IV dressing
- Tourniquet
- Gloves and apron

It's always worth **drawing up the saline flush** before cannulating as this is easier to do than when the cannula is *in situ*. If you're not experienced in cannulation it's worth taking a couple of spares in case you miss the first one.

Firstly **find the appropriate vein**. Selecting the best vein is important and you will learn this with practice. Essentially you want a large, straight vein which doesn't move around too much. Often these are ones that you cannot see directly but are obvious on palpation.

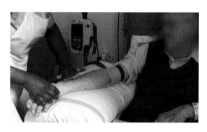

Select a suitable vein by first positioning the arm correctly and applying a tourniquet. Examine the whole of the area paying partiular attention to the back of the hand and the forearm

Small superficial veins are not ideal and in the elderly will probably last about 5 minutes if you manage to get a drip in.

In terms of vein selection, the veins on the **back of the hand** are the best to go for first. Although they can be more painful to put in (because the back of the hand is sensitive) they're comfortable once placed. They're easy to access, both for cannulation and for setting up a drip. And importantly, if the vein thromboses, you can always go more proximally later. Conversely if you thrombose a proximal vein, this can cause distal thrombosis as well – so it keeps your options open. When you've

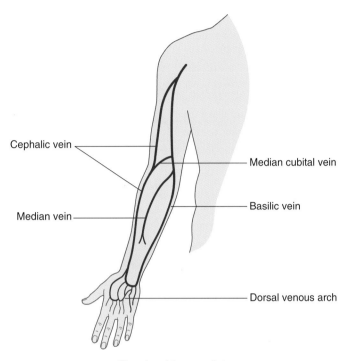

The veins of the upper limb

used these veins up, go to the forearm, for instance the 'houseman's' vein on the radial border of the forearm near the wrist, or the cephalic or basilic vein or one of their tributaries more proximally. Try to avoid veins that cross a joint, like in the antecubital fossa, where patients often complain of discomfort every time they bend their elbow. In an emergency situation you would however go straight for the antecubital fossa as the veins are bigger and easier to see.

However, in reality, most junior doctors go straight for the antecubital fossa because it's easier and because patients tend to complain that a needle in the back of the hand is painful. The nurses might not be too happy though as here the cannula tends to kink and set the pumps alarming. Remember also, to try and go for the non-dominant arm if possible.

Once you have selected your vein with careful palpation try and visualise exactly which direction it's running. **Place the tourniquet** about 4 finger widths above the cannulation site and ask the patient to **repeatedly clench and unclench** their fist. With a sterile alcohol based swab **clean the puncture site** and leave it 30 seconds to dry.

Remove the sheath from the cannula and '**unfurl' the wings**. The correct way to hold the cannula is with your forefinger and middlefinger on each wing and place your thumb over the end of the cannula. This way you can properly control the cannula as you advance it into the vein. If you remove the white cap you also tend to get a quicker flashback.

With your non-dominant hand **gently stretch the skin** over the vein to anchor it thus preventing it rolling from side to side, but not so firmly that it occludes.

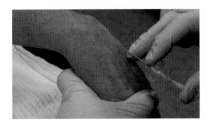

The cannula held in position ready to insert, the other hand secures the hand and gently stretches the skin

Warn the patient about a sharp scratch and **puncture the skin** at about 25° and look for a 'flashback' of blood into the cannula. With practice you may feel a slight give as the cannula enters the vein.

You will notice that the needle extends a few millimetres from the end of the cannula. This means that in practice once you achieve a flashback, the whole cannula and needle complex will need to be advanced a millimetre or so more before the needle can be withdrawn. Before you advance it **flatten the angle** with the skin to make it less acute, and when you **advance** try and follow exactly that mental image you had of the direction of where the vein is going.

Withdraw the needle about 3–4 mm keeping the plastic cannula still. This means that the needle is now hidden within the plastic cannula – your instrument of torture is now blunt but rigid. **Slide the whole complex into the vein** a few more millimetres. Advancing the cannula with the needle hidden inside is a great way of ensuring you stay in the vein.

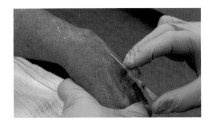

The cannula has entered the skin and flashback can be seen within it. Note the angle has now been reduced ready to advance

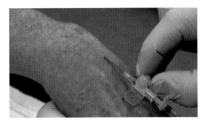

The needle is withdrawn slightly and the whole cannula, with partially withdrawn needle, is slowly advanced

Some people will, having got the needle into the vein, simultaneously advance the cannula whilst withdrawing the needle, however the cannula is pretty filimsy when not supported by the needle and can easily flick out of the vein.

Once inside by a few more millimetres, **withdraw the needle and advance the cannula. Release the tourniquet**, but press with your other hand on the proximal vein, otherwise when the needle comes out it will bleed everywhere. **Dispose immediately of your sharp** into a sharps bin.

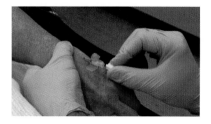

The needle is removed and pressure is applied proximally with the other hand to prevent bleeding. The white cap (that comes with the cannula) is about to be attached temporarily

Now at this point if you have been successful there will be blood pouring out of the cannula if you release your hand from the proximal vein. So **attach the connector** or the white cap that comes with every cannula.

Flush the cannula through the connector to ensure that the cannula doesn't clot off and to make sure that the flush is running easily into the vein without any pain or swelling.

Mop up any saline flush or blood and make sure the skin is **clean** and then **apply your dressing**. Nowadays many trusts have all-in-one cannula packs which will contain a special cannula-shaped adhesive dressing. These can be a bit tricky at first but generally work quite well. Make sure to stick the wings down first with the small bits of tape that come with it. Often an extra bit of tape placed horizontally across the top is useful to stop the cannula catching on anything. Be sure, however, that only transparent adhesive dressing covers the actual entry point through the skin. This allows visual inspection for signs of phlebitis. **Dispose of your waste**.

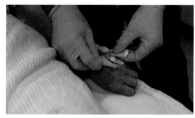

A standard cannula dressing is applied; be sure not to cover up the skin where the cannula actually enters – this is the first place you check for phlebitis

All that remains is some **documentation**. All cannulas now need to be recorded for how long they have been in for. This is usually done on the cannula itself with a small sticker with the date when it was sited. Many trusts now have gone even further and developed 'saving lives' sheets or cannula 'care plans'. Basically this is a sheet of paper that goes in the observation folder and documents when the cannula went in, what type it was, where it was sited and when it should come out. The nurses also check and document for any signs of phlebitis. Regardless of this all cannulae generally are removed after 3 days as a precaution. In addition in some trusts there will be a small sticker which is enclosed with the cannula which needs to be signed and stuck in the notes. Yes … this may all seems a bit of a hassle but infection control is considered very important these days – it's worth doing your bit of the paperwork or you will get in trouble.

Finally you may need to remove a cannula. This is usually if it's no longer required or there is phlebitis present. This is pretty straightforward: After washing your hands and putting on some gloves, peel off the dressing and then withdraw the cannula whilst covering the puncture site with gauze. Give some gentle pressure and secure the gauze in place for a few hours.

Remember – when you're doing your ward-round just think: is this cannula really needed? They might seem harmless but they can be an avoidable source of potentially life threatening infection!

OSCE checklist

- Assembles equipment correctly
- Draws up flush
- Flushes connector
- Positions arm correctly and places tourniquet
- Selects suitable vein
- Cleans site
- Warns about a 'sharp scratch'
- Inserts IV cannula at about 15–30°
- Observes for flashback of dark venous blood
- Partially withdraws needle keeping sheath still
- Advances cannula (with needle partially withdrawn)
- Releases tourniquet
- Manually compresses vein proximally
- Withdraws needle and disposes into sharps bin
- Attaches connector and flushes
- Secures with dressing
- Places review date sticker
- Completes cannula insertion sticker and places in clinical notes
- Washes hands
- Thanks patient
- Documents procedure
- Provides postprocedure advice

32 Pleural Aspiration

| Video Time | 2 mins 41 s |

Overview

A pleural tap (or in north America *needle thoracocentesis*) is a simple, but invasive test to sample fluid from around the lung. This is almost always done as a **diagnostic test** when a patient has a **unilateral pleural effusion**. Other liquids can accumulate around the lung, for example blood (haemothorax) or pus (empyema) however in these cases the fluid is usually removed with an **intercostal (chest) drain** (see Chapters 23: Large Bore Chest Drain and 34: Seldinger Chest Drain).

Bilateral effusions are generally **not** tapped. This is because bilateral effusions tend to be due to a systemic organ failure leading to a transudative effusion (for example heart failure, cirrhosis or nephrotic syndrome). In these cases there is little diagnostic value of a tap and treatment is directed at the underlying cause. The British Thoracic Society (BTS) does however recommend tapping bilateral effusions if there are atypical features, or the patient does not respond to therapy.

Why perform a pleural tap? We can discover much about the aetiology of an effusion by fluid analysis. As with other '3rd space' fluids (such as ascites) we can divide them into transudates and exudates. As we all remember, transudates occur due to an imbalance in the fluid hydrostatic and oncotic pressures leading to fluid shift into non-physiological third spaces. Transudates typically have a **low** protein content of <25 g/L and are caused by the 'failures' – heart, renal and liver. These typically lead to bilateral effusions. Exudates on the other hand typically occur due to an inflammatory or malignant process causing fluid to 'exude' from the vasculature. They typically have **higher** protein counts >25 g/L and result in unilateral effusions.

How to Perform Clinical Procedures, First Edition. Matthew Stephenson, Joshua Shur and John Black.
© 2013 John Wiley & Sons, Ltd. Published 2013 by John Wiley & Sons, Ltd.

Indications	(Relative) Contraindications	Complications
• Investigation of unilateral pleural effusion • Investigation of bilateral pleural effusion with atypical features or not responding to treatment	• Infection at site of tap • Uncorrected bleeding diathesis • Small amount of fluid, unlikely to be tapped • Mechanical ventilation	• Bleeding • Infection • Pneumothorax • Haemopneumothorax • Cough • Damage to intercostal neurovascular bundle

As a junior, particularly if you are on a respiratory or acute medicine firm you will encounter plenty of patients requiring a tap and for this reason it's a very **important skill to learn**. It is a relatively straightforward procedure, particularly since the advent of ultrasound.

Procedure

Pleural tap was traditionally a 'blind' procedure, but now most commonly is done using ultrasound guidance.

Ultrasound can be used to image the procedure in 'real-time', or to identify the location of fluid beforehand. The BTS states that thoracic ultrasound guidance is strongly recommended for all pleural procedures – and if facilities exist and you have been properly trained you should use it.

If you have proper training you can locate the fluid yourself, or you can ask a radiologist to do it for you. If marking the site beforehand, the BTS recommend that this should only be done for large effusions. Typically after the fluid is located, a mark is left for where to aim for.

Sometimes there might be more complicated collections (for example loculated or septated) which need tapping and in these cases it is better to use ultrasound – if this is the case, it should be done by a radiologist or someone with appropriate training in ultrasound – so almost certainly not you.

Ultrasound is more sensitive than a plain chest x-ray for locating smaller effusions. A chest x-ray taken supine may make it even more difficult to locate fluid (for example in a trauma case). We won't go into all the details for how to locate fluid with ultrasound as specific training is required, but in a nutshell the intercostal space is imaged in real time and black anechoic fluid is located in between lung and diaphragm. It is important to recognise that the pleural space will change in dimensions with respiration. You can also measure the rough distance required that you will need to insert the needle during the procedure.

There is some evidence that performing the procedure with real-time ultrasonography can reduce the rate of pneumothorax.

Make sure you have the **correct patient**, for this procedure. Check for any **allergies**, and that you have confirmed the **indication;** excluded any **contraindications** (particularly for instance warfarin therapy, the BTS advises to perform an elective tap only if the INR is <1.5); **explained** the procedure and taken **consent**. Now **wash your hands**!

Examine your patient and make sure you are confident where the effusion is. The next crucial step is to **review their imaging**, and for this you **must** have a good chest x-ray. Once this confirms our suspicions of an effusion we are ready to proceed.

Assemble all of your equipment on a trolley. You will need everything in the equipment textbox.

Equipment you need (on a sterile tray/trolley)

- 50 ml syringe for sample
- 10 ml syringe for local anaesthetic
- Green needle
- Gauze
- Skin-prep solution
- Sterile gloves
- Specimen containers
- Local anaesthetic
- 10 ml syringe
- Blue and green needles to infiltrate anaesthetic
- Bedside ultrasound probe with sterile probe cover and sterile acoustic gel (if necessary)

Position your patient sat **upright** (make sure they don't have a nap immediately beforehand as we want gravity to draw all that fluid towards the ground!) and have them rest their arms comfortably, for example on a table.

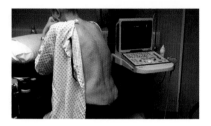

Patient seated upright with their back exposed. Have their arms resting comfortably on a table or trolley

Auscultate and percuss down the posterior chest until you have found the upper border of the effusion. Our tap site will be 1 or 2 rib spaces below this. Remember to avoid the scapula, at least 2 inches should be enough. If it has not been done already – **mark the skin**. Note that this may be a different place to where you might insert a chest drain. If you are using ultrasound, image in the intercostal space to confirm the presence of fluid. **Most people would advocate tapping from the safe triangle if fluid is there**. It is

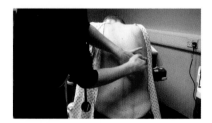

Percussing over the back to confirm the position of the effusion

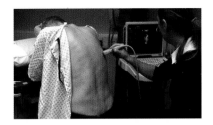

Positioning the ultrasound probe in the intercostal space to confirm location of fluid

also important to note that closer to the spine the neurovascular bundle can dip lower making the procedure potentially more risky.

Wash your hands again and put on your **sterile gloves, and ideally a sterile gown**. Take your skin-prep solution and liberally **clean the area**. Make sure to allow it to dry if you are using an alcohol based cleaning solution.

We are hoping for a decent amount of fluid and the guidelines recommend a **50 ml syringe** should be enough. Attach this to a **green needle** and you

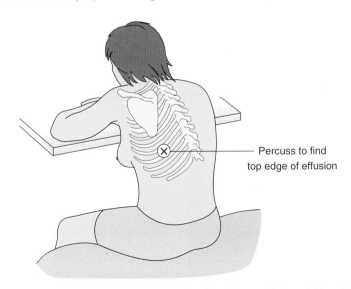

Percuss to find top edge of effusion

Percuss over the back for the upper edge of dullness. It's sensible to mark this out are good-to-go. If you are going to use local anaesthetic then this is the time to infiltrate. As always, start with a bleb at the surface and then infiltrate the deeper structures aiming for a tract that your needle will pass through. Particularly make sure to aspirate first and be sure to avoid the neurovascular bundle which sits in a groove at the inferior aspect of the rib above, therefore always aim for 'above the rib below, not below the rib above'. You will know that you have infiltrated far enough when you aspirate fluid – indicating that you have entered the pleural space.

Aim just **above** the rib below and insert your needle **perpendicular to the skin**. **Advance the needle** slowly, aspirating on the syringe as you do so. You should start to receive fluid as soon as the tip of the needle enters the pleural cavity – **take a 50 ml syringe-full**. **Remove your needle** and apply some gauze and a suitable dressing. The procedure itself is as simple as that – as with many procedures, it's the decision-making and preparation that's key. Put a

suitable simple **dressing** over the site.

Ensure your samples are **correctly labelled** and that the **request form has been fully completed**. Finally as always, **document** your procedure. Along with all the essentials (date, time etc.) document how much local was used, if you used ultrasound first, whether it was a straight-forward procedure or not and what tests you sent for. Also document that consent was obtained. In general, for simple pleural aspiration a chest x-ray is not required

---

Therapeutic pleural tap

So far we have discussed *diagnostic* taps, but occasionally the procedure can be modified if it's to be done as a *therapeutic* tap. Essentially if a patient is breathless or in discomfort we would prefer to get the fluid off entirely. This does of course run the risk of re-accumulation and if this does occur then a chest drain may be necessary.

To entirely remove an effusion we use a 3-way tap with a 50 ml syringe. A green-needle really isn't big enough to do the job, so we tend to use a grey cannula.

The procedure is briefly described: Once the cannula is in the pleural space, remove the needle and attach the cannula to a 3-way tap. When the cannula is in place make sure you don't give your patient a pneumothorax so put your finger over the end. Using your syringe you can repeatedly aspirate and discard the pleural fluid into a container.

As the fluid is removed and the lung re-expands the pleura tends to get a little irritated as the pleura touches the tip of your cannula and the patient will likely start to cough. Warn the patient of this. The BTS recommends that after 1.5L the procedure should be stopped, or when the patient starts to cough.

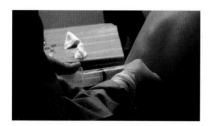

Successful aspiration of pleural fluid

postprocedure.

Now you have done your procedure you have to decide what to do with your sample. Have a **look at the fluid** – is it purulent or clear? Blood stained or not? All of these will give you some clues as to its aetiology.

The BTS recommend a plethora of tests to send the fluid for (see below) and if you are going to look at **Light's criteria** (see later) then make sure you send off a paired blood sample too.

Tests to send for:
- Protein
- LDH
- Gram stain and culture ('M, C+S')
- Cytology: the BTS note that a lymphocyte predominance tends to be typical of malignancy, heart failure and TB. This won't give you your diagnosis but can help narrow down the differential
- Paired blood sample for total protein and LDH

'Other' tests:
- pH: the BTS recommend this where infection is suspected but that tap is non-purulent. In addition if there is a parapneumonic effusion with a pH <7.2 then you will need to drain it with an intercostal drain. Be careful though, if the tap is frankly purulent then it could damage a gas machine
- Amylase: occasionally a unilateral effusion may be associated with pancreatic disease or oesophageal rupture. In these cases an amylase may be useful

---

Light's criteria

Light defined a set of criteria to distinguish between an exudative and transudative effusion. These are not only useful, but will impress on a ward round if you know them! Essentially an effusion is exudative if:
- The ratio of pleural fluid protein to serum protein is greater than 0.5
- The ratio of pleural fluid LDH and serum LDH is greater than 0.6
- Pleural fluid LDH is greater than two-thirds the normal upper limit for serum.

So to calculate it you will need both sample and serum LDH and protein (i.e. a paired sample)

OSCE checklist

- Assembles equipment correctly
- Seats patient with back exposed
- Confirms dullness to percussion
- Locates fluid using ultrasound (optional)
- Holds ultrasound probe in intercostal space
- Marks position
- Assembles equipment correctly
- Dons sterile gloves (and optional gown)
- Cleans area
- Places 'inco' pad (optional)
- Checks and draws up local anaesthetic
- Warns about a 'sharp scratch'
- Infiltrates local anaesthetic correctly
- Inserts needle perpendicular to rib
- Advances needle slowly whilst aspirating
- Aspirates sample successfully

- Removes needle and applies pressure with gauze
- Applies appropriate dressing
- Labels samples and completes request form correctly
- Washes hands
- Thanks patient
- Disposes of sharps and waste
- Documents procedure
- Provides postprocedure advice

33 Ring Block

Video Time | 1 min 56 s

Overview

Considering humans use their fingers (and to a lesser extent their toes) for so many everyday functions, it's not surprising that they should come into trouble now and again. A laceration on a broken glass, an avulsion of the tip or even a full-blown digital amputation. These injuries will come to find you in A&E. On the toes, the most common problem is an ingrown toenail, but the same injuries can present there too.

The marvelous thing about digital trauma is how easy it is to numb the affected area. If you had to inject local anaesthetic directly into the affected area, this would be extremely painful since the skin of the fingers is so sensitive, plus the subcutaneous layer is tight, making local infiltration more difficult. On each side of the digit are digital nerves. Without getting bogged down with the derivation of these nerves, put simply there is a digital nerve running up the lateral border and another running up the medial border of each finger or toe. If you anaesthetise the nerves proximally, close to the base of the digit, the whole digit becomes completely numb.

Indications	Contraindications	Complications
• Local anaesthesia before any painful procedure on a digit	• Compromised digital circulation, e.g. severe Raynauds • Local infection at the puncture site	• Nil of note

How to Perform Clinical Procedures, First Edition. Matthew Stephenson, Joshua Shur and John Black.
© 2013 John Wiley & Sons, Ltd. Published 2013 by John Wiley & Sons, Ltd.

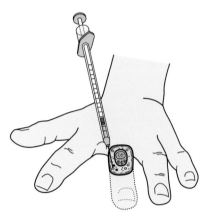

The digital nerves run up the side of each finger

Procedure

Make sure you have the **correct patient**, for the **correct procedure**. Check for any **allergies**, and that you have confirmed the **indication;** excluded any **contraindications; explained** the procedure and taken **consent**. Now **wash your hands**!

Assemble all of your equipment on a sterile trolley away from the patient. You will need everything in the equipment textbox.

It's usually easiest to have the patient's hand **flat on a hard surface** like a table, palm down. **Clean the skin** of the finger and adjacent part of the hand. It may be best not to clean the laceration itself (assuming that's why you're doing the block) until the finger is numb as this can really sting. Depending on what you're doing the block for you will probably also need to **create a sterile field** around the finger using a sterile drape.

Here's one of the most important parts: **NEVER USE LOCAL ANAESTHETIC WITH ADRENALINE IN A RING BLOCK**. Adrenaline can be great for use with local anaesthesia in other areas as it increases the dose of local you can use without cardiotoxicity (see above, Chapter 25: Local Anaesthetic Infiltration); however, in the fingers and toes these are end arteries – that is, you will render the digit ischaemic. The truth is, the digit will probably survive the insult as the adrenaline will wear off before too long, but don't put it to the test.

Draw up the local anaesthetic into the 10 ml syringe with the 21G needle and replace with your 23G or 25G needle. **Expel any air** from the syringe.

Warn the patient about a **sharp scratch. Insert the needle perpendicular** to the skin as proximally as you can go, close to the web space on the dorsal surface. **Aim** for just to the side of the proximal part of the proximal phalanx. Keep **advancing the needle slowly**, you're hoping to just glide past the bone. If you hit the bone, the patient won't thank you as it will be very painful (periosteum is very sensitive), just withdraw slightly and re-aim slightly away from the bone. Equally you don't want to be too superficial.

Keep **advancing the needle** slowly past the bone and **watch on the palmar side** of the finger to see a tiny bulge where the needle is getting close to coming all the way through the finger. **Stop here**. Don't let the needle go all the way through the finger, there's no value in anaesthetising the table. **Slowly withdraw** the needle whilst **gently pressing** on the syringe. You are aiming to distribute about 1–2 ml (depending on the thickness of the finger) along the track of your needle on the way back out. **Repeat** exactly the same thing on the other side of the finger. You can then go on to complete whatever procedure you were planning.

Notes

Some people advocate **aspirating** the syringe before injecting. This is perfectly OK too, the rationale is that you don't want to inject local into an artery. However, the digital arteries are tiny vessels, if you are slowly withdrawing your needle and injecting as you go, even if the tip does pass through the artery on the way back out it will be in it for a miniscule fraction of a second especially considering how much it will spasm in response to the trauma of the needle.

Bear in mind also that some people put in the ring block even more proximally, especially for the toes. You can actually do a toe amputation for instance under ring block by instead of going at the level of the web spaces, passing the needle between the contiguous metatarsals, that is, through the dorsum of the foot.

OSCE checklist
- Assembles equipment correctly
- Checks local anaesthetic
- Draws up local anaesthetic correctly
- Cleans injection site
- Inserts needle on lateral side of digit
- Advances through most of digit
- Withdraws whilst infiltrating about 2 mls
- Repeats on other side of digit
- Checks effectiveness before proceeding further
- Performs intended procedure
- Washes hands
- Thanks patient
- Disposes of sharps and waste
- Documents procedure
- Provides postprocedure advice

34 Seldinger Chest Drain

Joy Edlin and Michael Marrinan

Video Time | 9 mins 17 s

Overview

When it comes to chest drains, you've got two main options: a **large bore** (24–30 F) intercostal chest drain inserted by an **open technique** (see Chapter 23: Large Bore Chest Drain) or a **narrow bore** (8–14 F) drain inserted using the **Seldinger technique**. Broadly speaking, surgeons tend to do the former and medics the latter. This is because large bore chest drains are needed for draining blood (which can be viscous) resulting from trauma or surgery, whereas narrow bore chest drains are good for low viscosity 'medical' pleural effusions. Pneumothoraces can be drained by either, but air tends to escape more easily and with less resistance from a large bore drain. There are other instances where either type of drain may be appropriate, but just remember to consider whether what you're draining is likely to block a narrow tube. Performing a **diagnostic pleural tap** first may help with this choice. Thick viscous pus, for instance, will need a big drain.

There will be quite a bit of repetition here from Chapter 23– but these are points worth labouring.

This is a pretty straightforward procedure to perform, but with 'superspecialisation' is increasingly being performed by certain specialties only. State to seniors early on that you wish to learn to do it, so they think of you when the opportunity arises.

Procedure

Make sure you have the **correct patient**, for the **correct procedure**. Check for any **allergies**, and that you have confirmed the **indication;** excluded any **contraindications; explained** the procedure

How to Perform Clinical Procedures, First Edition. Matthew Stephenson, Joshua Shur and John Black.
© 2013 John Wiley & Sons, Ltd. Published 2013 by John Wiley & Sons, Ltd.

Indications	Contraindications	Complications

• Hydrothorax
  ◦ Effusion (low
    protein content)
  ◦ Low viscosity
    empyema
• Spontaneous
  pneumothorax
	• Refractory coagulopathy
	• Infection in overlying skin/soft tissues
	• Lung densely adherent to chest wall
	• Relative contraindications:
	  ◦ Loculated effusion – likely to require
	    drainage under ultrasound or CT
	    guidance
	  ◦ Pleural scarring (thickening)
	  ◦ Presence of diaphragmatic hernia
		• Pneumothorax/
		  tension
		  pneumothorax
		• Haemothorax
		• Bleeding
		• Infection
		• Injury to solid
		  organs

and taken **consent**, which in some trusts needs to be in the written form for a chest drain. Now **wash your hands**!

Assemble all of your equipment on a sterile trolley away from the patient. You will need everything in the equipment textbox. Make sure you have an **assistant** throughout, they will need to hand you things as you will be sterile, and they will also need to connect the drain to the drainage bottle.

Set up the equipment trolley and **prepare your closed drainage system** with the underwater seal. The latter is formed by adding sterile water to your collection bottle up to the premarked

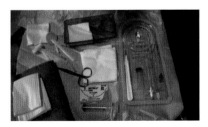

The equipment laid out on a sterile trolley

Equipment you need (on a sterile tray/trolley)

- 'Your' equipment
  - Face mask
  - Sterile gown
  - Sterile gloves
  - Surgical hat to cover hair
- Procedure equipment
  - Dressing pack or chest drain insertion pack which includes:
    - Sterile cover for trolley
    - Gauze swabs
    - Gallipot or tub for skin prep
  - Seldinger chest drain kit, incl. chest drain (usually 10–14 F)
  - Scalpel/blade
  - Sterile drapes
  - Skin prep
  - Connecting tubing
  - Closed drainage system allowing underwater seal
  - Sterile water
  - Local anaesthetic (e.g., 10 ml 1% lidocaine)
  - 10 ml syringe for the local anaesthetic
  - Green needle (21G)
  - Blue needle (23G)
  - Suture, e.g. 1 silk with large curved needle
  - Sterile scissors
  - Dressing

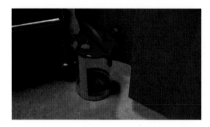

The chest drain bottle prefilled with water up to the mark

line. This creates a one-way valve, which allows air out of the pleural space, but prevents air getting in.

Ensure radiographic images are available. It's now **mandatory to have three-dimensional imaging** of the chest before chest drain insertion in the form of either a **CT or ultrasound** (yes we know that's 2D, but as soon as you move the probe around it gives you a 3D understanding), except in dire emergencies.

Examine the patient. This will help you confirm the indication and side, and identify the necessary **anatomical landmarks** as well as help demarcate the **fluid or air level**.

Your anatomical landmarks are:
- **5th intercostal space** (ICS)
- **Anterior axillary line** (immediately lateral to the lateral border of pectoralis major)
- The literature quotes the **safe triangle of insertion** as bordered by the lateral side of the pectoralis major muscle anteriorly, the anterior border of latissimus dorsi posteriorly, the axilla apically and a line along the 5th ICS/through the nipple

inferiorly. These borders should be viewed with caution as the anterior border of latissimus dorsi actually lies behind the midaxillary line and you *must* insert the drain anterior to the midaxillary line.

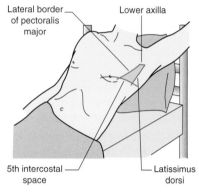

The safe triangle

Position the patient **resting at 45°** with the arm on the affected side resting over their head. This allows you free access to the site and stretches the chest wall opening up the rib spaces. Alternatively, the patient can sit upright leaning over a pillow.

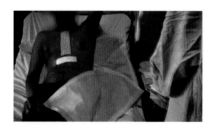

The patient positioned to stretch out the chest wall

Identify your **anatomical landmarks** again and **mark the site**, where you deem it safe to insert the drain.

Now you can **scrub** and don your sterile **protective clothing**. **Clean** the site with skin preparation. **Drape** the patient, leaving only the site and its immediate surroundings exposed. An aperture drape is ideal for this as it has a hole in the middle which can be aligned with the planned drainage site.

Prepare to **infiltrate local anaesthetic** (LA) into the site. When inserting the needle, remember to aim for the top of the 6th rib, but before you hit it deviate upwards slightly, so that the **needle rests on top of the rib**. This avoids damage to the intercostal neurovascular bundle. Gently pass the needle through the tissues, whilst applying constant negative pressure on the syringe, until you enter the pleura. If you're able to easily **aspirate** fluid or air into your syringe you know it's safe to proceed. If you're unable to aspirate fluid it's unsafe for you to place the drain here. You should then **ask for help** from a more senior member of your team. If you're experienced, however, you may attempt to insert the drain along the posterior axillary line instead. If in any doubt, it's better to insert a chest drain under ultrasound guidance.

Once positive aspiration has confirmed a safe drain position, **infiltrate the tissues**, with LA. Leave this to work its magic for a couple of minutes. Confirm that the tissues are numb before you **make a small nick in the skin** using a blade.

Now, let's talk about this Seldinger chest drain kit. It comprises most importantly:
- a **bevelled needle**
- a **guide wire**
- a **dilator**
- the **chest drain** itself

So first, here's a spoiler of how the **Seldinger technique** works: the needle will be inserted into the pleural cavity, then the guide wire will be threaded through the needle allowing the needle to be removed without losing one's position and entrance into the pleura. This guide wire is the central core of the Seldinger technique, and is the same principle applied to central venous lines, angiograms, etc. Essentially it provides something to railroad catheters, sheaths, balloons, etc. through. A dilator will then be passed to create a track through the tissues and finally the drain will be passed over the guide wire and the guide wire can be removed.

Attach the 10 ml **syringe** to the graded and bevelled needle in the kit and **insert the needle**, bevelled edge up, through the tissues in the same direction that your local anaesthetic needle went, aspirating gently as you proceed. Remember to aim your needle **above the 6th rib**, rather than below the 5th rib. This is to avoid the neurovascular bundle that runs on the undersurface of the rib. Once you enter the pleura you will once again aspirate fluid, confirming your position. This fluid can be sent for various investigations required. Make a note of how deep you had to pass the needle through the chest wall – this tells you how deep the pleural cavity is under the skin. This is important for later.

Anchor the needle with one hand and remove the syringe with the other, so the needle is still in position. With your free hand pass the guide wire through the needle, ensuring you **never let go of the guide wire**, until about 20 cm of the wire (there are markings on the wire) have been threaded through. Without ever letting go of the guide wire, **remove the needle** so just the guide wire is going through the track. Now **pass the dilator** over the guide wire and through the tissues to create a passage for the drain. This is why it was important to make a note of how far you had to put the needle in: **you should only insert the dilator as far as the**

needle went, which may just be 3 or 4 centimetres. This can be a dangerous bit of equipment if inserted fully, there have been disastrous cases of it entering the left atrium. The dilator should pass easily. If it doesn't, you haven't made the nick in the skin deep enough (because it won't dilate skin well, just the deeper tissues) or the guide wire is kinked. **Remove the dilator**.

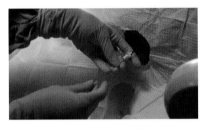

The guidewire is being threaded through the needle

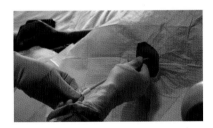

The dilator is threaded over the guidewire

Now you can **pass the chest drain** over the wire. The drain has a small stiff plastic piece inside it, which helps maintain the curve at the business end. Keep this piece in to help maintain this curvature and direct the drain around and behind the ribs, aiming inferoposteriorly in the pleural space for a hydrothorax or apically if there's a pneumothorax. Bear in mind, however, that this sounds fine in theory, but actually Seldinger drains are pretty undirectable unlike a large bore chest drain. If it gets in to the right place it was probably more by good fortune than skill.

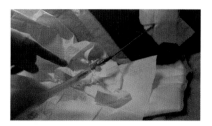

The tubing is connected to the drain via a 3-way tap here

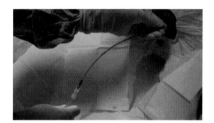

The chest drain itself is threaded over the guidewire

The length of the drain is marked along its course. How far you insert it depends on the depth of the effusion and the body habitus of the patient. You should insert the drain to **at least 10–12 cm**.

When you're confident it's in the right place, **remove the guide wire** followed by the **stiff inner plastic piece**. Place a **closed 3-way tap** on the end of the drain to **avoid the introduction of air**. Secure the drain in place with a **stay suture**, **connect** it to the underwater seal via the connecting tubing and **open the 3-way tap** to release the effusion. You don't need to insert a horizontal mattress suture as with a large bore chest drain since the hole is only small and will close spontaneously by elastic recoil.

Simple suture to secure the drain with the anchoring knot near the point of fixation to the drain

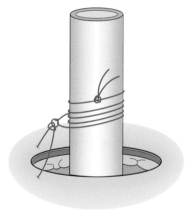

Stay suture – tethering to the skin and a tight sling around the drain

Clean and dress the site, making sure that it's airtight around the tube and arrange a **chest x-ray to exclude a pneumothorax**. Confirmation of the position of the drain is less important as the fluid will continue to drain varying with the position of the patient. If the chest x-ray reveals a new pneumothorax, the drain should be placed on negative suction to aid removal of the air and re-expansion of the lung.

Dispose of your sharps directly into a sharps bin and your waste into a clinical waste bin. **Wash your hands** and **record the procedure** clearly in the patient's notes.

OSCE checklist

- Confirms indication on 3D imaging
- Identifies the chest wall landmarks
- Identifies site for drain in 4th or 5th intercostal space
- Confirms correct side on examination
- Washes hands and dons sterile gloves and gown
- Assembles equipment correctly
- Checks local anaesthetic
- Positions patient appropriately
- Cleans skin appropriately
- Creates sterile field
- Reconfirms position for drain placement
- Warns about a 'sharp scratch'
- Raises a bleb of local under the skin
- Infiltrates local anaesthetic to deep layers
- Understands the Seldinger technique
- Tests the effect of the local anaesthetic
- Makes a small stab incision
- Inserts the needle introducer
- Successfully aspirates pleural fluid
- Threads guidewire
- Always keeps hold of the guidewire
- Removes needle
- Threads the dilator over the guidewire
- Removes the dilator
- Threads the chest drain over the wire
- Removes the guidewire
- Removes the stiff inner tube from the chest drain
- Connects the 3-way port
- Attaches the tubing adaptor
- Secures the drain
- Asks assistant to connect one end of the tubing to the bottle
- Connects the tubing to the chest drain
- Fashions an airtight padded dressing
- Confirms final position by assessing 'swing'
- Requests chest x-ray to confirm position
- Washes hands
- Thanks patient
- Disposes of sharps and waste
- Documents procedure
- Provides postprocedure advice

35 Spinal Injection

Vanessa Fludder

Video Time | 4 mins 13 s

Overview

Spinal anaesthesia is used to anaesthetise (cause 'numbness') the lower part of the body and can be used for operations below the umbilicus. It is also known as a 'subarachnoid' or 'intrathecal' block. Many terms, same thing.

Spinal anaesthesia is commonly used for hip/knee replacement surgery and can be used for most operations on the lower limbs. Its use is limited by the duration of anaesthesia provided by a spinal anaesthetic, which is usually around 2 hours. It's the most common form of anaesthesia used for caesarean sections as it avoids side-effects of general anaesthesia for both mother and baby. If the procedure is likely to last longer than 2 hours then a combined spinal and epidural would be more appropriate as the epidural catheter can be used to top up the anaesthesia as it starts to wear off.

There are not many absolute contraindications to performing spinal anaesthesia, patient refusal being just about the only absolute contraindication. Raised ICP is an obvious contraindication. If in doubt, always ask.

Abnormal clotting poses a risk of epidural haematoma, which is a rare but very serious complication. Before doing a spinal, a full blood count should be done to confirm a platelet count of > 100. If the platelet count is less than 100 a clotting screen is required. Ordinarily a patient with an INR or APTR of greater than 1.5 should not receive a spinal. Most anaesthetists would not perform a spinal on a patient taking clopidogrel unless it has been stopped for at least 5 days. A patient on prophylactic heparin/LMWH should not have a spinal injection within 12 hours of the last dose, or 24 hours if on a fully anticoagulant treatment dose. Similar precautions need to be taken when a patient is receiving any oral anticoagulant, you should look up the particular time constraints for the particular drug in question.

How to Perform Clinical Procedures, First Edition. Matthew Stephenson, Joshua Shur and John Black.
© 2013 John Wiley & Sons, Ltd. Published 2013 by John Wiley & Sons, Ltd.

Indications	Contraindications	Complications
• Regional anaesthesia for surgery to lower limbs, caesarean section.	• Raised ICP • Coagulopathy (relative – see below) • Spina bifida	• Motor blockade of legs • Urinary retention • Post Dural Puncture Headache (PDPH) • Meningitis (rare) • Epidural haematoma (rare) • Epidural abscess (rare) • Paralysis (rare)

A history of spina bifida would deter most anaesthetists due to the possibility of damaging a tethered low-lying cord. An MRI can be done to demonstrate the anatomy and position of the cord.

One needs to be very careful when performing a spinal in anyone with a relatively fixed cardiac output (i.e. unable to increase stroke volume and heart rate in response to a fall in systemic vascular resistance). For example, anyone with severe aortic or mitral stenosis should have an arterial line and very close monitoring/manipulation of blood pressure if a spinal is thought to be the best (least worst) option for anaesthesia. A combined spinal/epidural is often the safest (haemodynamically stable) option.

Complications

The local anaesthetic used to provide anaesthesia also causes a motor block. Thus the legs usually become heavy and immobile. A urinary catheter is usually inserted as the patient is unable to sense a full bladder and/or void successfully. It's common to use a combination of both a local anaesthetic and an opioid in a spinal injection. The latter provides better, more prolonged analgesia but causes an all over itchy prickly feeling which may last for up to 24 hours after the anaesthetic has worn off.

Most patients having a spinal which spreads up to thoracic dermatomes will have a degree of hypotension caused by sympathetic blockade. Generally the degree of hypotension is greater the higher the level of block. It is usually easily treated with small intermittent boluses of a vasopressor such as phenylephrine, metaraminol or ephedrine. It's essential to have good wide bore venous access before giving a spinal anaesthetic in order to rapidly correct (with vasopressors and fluids) any hypotension which may occur. The drop in blood pressure can be quite dramatic, especially in pregnancy.

Serious complications are unusual. Depending on the size of the needle used, a Post Dural Puncture Headache (PDPH) may ensue. Anaesthetists use spinal needles which are very fine, in the order of 24–27 g, contrasting with the 20/22 g needles often used to perform an LP. The risk of a PDPH when using a 24 g or smaller atraumatic needle is about 1 in 500. Most PDP headaches will resolve spontaneously within a week. The smaller the needle, the smaller the risk of a headache. The risk of headache is also reduced by using a rounded tipped needle with the hole on the side rather than a cutting tip with the hole at the end.

Very serious complications are exceedingly rare. Possible complications include meningitis, epidural haematoma, epidural abscess, paralysis. According to the 3rd Anaesthetic National Audit Project the risk of permanent harm or death after a peri-operative spinal anaesthetic is 1 in 38 462.

Procedure

Make sure you have the **correct patient**, for the **correct procedure**. Check for any **allergies**, and that you have confirmed the **indication;** excluded any **contraindications; explained** the procedure and taken **consent**. Now **wash your hands**!

Assemble all of your equipment on a sterile trolley away from the patient. You will need everything in the equipment textbox.

The procedure must be done in a **sterile** manner which means a proper scrub-up and the wearing of a hat, mask, sterile gown and sterile gloves. The patient's skin should be decontaminated with 0.5% chlorhexidine (which must not come into contact with any needles or equipment in your sterile tray as it's neurotoxic) and allowed to dry.

> **Equipment you need (on a sterile trolley)**
>
> - Sterile gown, surgical hat and mask
> - Sterile gloves
> - Antiseptic cleaning solution e.g. chlorhexidine 0.5%
> - Injectate for establishing anaesthesia (see following table (The different typical injectates and patient positions for some specific procedures)
> - Sterile aperture drape
> - Introducer needle
> - Spinal needle
> - Syringe
> - Something cold to test anaesthesia (e.g. cold spray/ice cube)
> - Simple dressing if required

Decide which **position** would be preferable depending on the area you want to anaesthetise (see below). If either position is acceptable ask your patient which they would find more comfortable. If they choose to sit you should ask them to '**slouch**' for you, as this will optimise the curvature of their lumbar spine and open up the spaces between the spinous processes. If your patient might be more comfortable in the lateral position, ask them to curl up like a hedgehog/woodlouse.

If you are using 'heavy bupivacaine' and the operative procedure is to be performed on the right leg, for example, your patient will be better off lying on their right-hand side, with the left leg uppermost. The spread of 'heavy' bupivacaine can be directed by gravity, whereas plain bupivacaine cannot.

Identify the landmarks. Usually one should aim for L2/3 or L3/4. The spinal cord usually ends somewhere around T12–L1, so below L2 should be safe and well away from the spinal cord.

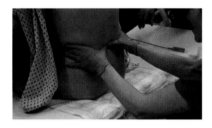

Palpating the level of the iliac crests in the midline

Place a **sterile drape** with a hole in the middle over the patients back. Aim to place the hole in the centre of the back approximately level with the iliac crest. **Feel** for the inter-spinous space at this level and use some lidocaine to numb

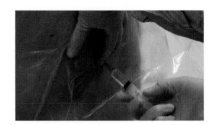

Infiltrating local anaesthetic into the deeper tissues before inserting the introducer

the skin and sub-cutaneous tissue at your entry point. You will need to use an 'introducer needle' when using fine gauge pencil point spinal needles as they are too flimsy and not sharp enough to penetrate the skin. A pencil point needle is unlikely to damage neural tissue.

Draw up your injectate. It's likely that this will be some bupivacaine mixed with an opiate such as diamorphine or fentanyl.

Introduce your introducer needle in the midline, in the middle of the space you can feel between two spinous processes. Aim roughly horizontal, and if your needle encounters bone withdraw a bit and aim a little more cephalad. If you hit bone again, withdraw and aim a little more cephalad, repeat until your passage is clear. When you are (on average) about 6–7 cm deep you might feel a little give, like a small pop. **Remove the stylet** from the spinal needle and if you are in the correct place CSF will flow back into the needle hub and start to drip out slowly. **Attach your syringe** with your intended injectate. **Aspirate**. You should see CSF swirling as it mixes with your injectate in the syringe. **Inject**. In general the faster you inject, the more it will spread. When you have finished **remove both needles**; there isn't usually any need to cover the tiny hole, but you can use a small dressing if you wish.

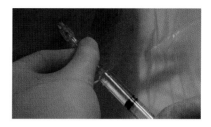

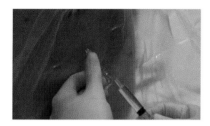

Attaching syringe of injectate to spinal needle and introducer before aspirating CSF to confirm correct placement

If you are aiming for just a saddle block, anaesthetising just sacral dermatomes, leave the patient in the sitting position for a few minutes before laying the patient down. If the patient is having a caesarean section, the numbness will need to extend up to about T4 so you will need to lie your patient down to allow the heavy bupivacaine to spread with gravity.

The different typical injectates and patient positions for some specific procedures

Type of surgery	Suitable injectate	Position	Spread
Caesarean section	0.5% heavy bupivacaine (2.2–2.7 mls) + 300 mcg diamorphine	Lateral or sitting position	Needs to spread up to T4
Perineal tear/ haemorrhoidectomy	0.5% heavy bupivacaine 1.5 mls (+/- fentanyl 10–20 mcg)	Sitting	Sacral dermatomes
TURP/TURBT	0.5% heavy bupivacaine (2.5–3 mls) + 300 mcg diamorphine or 15 mcg fentanyl	Sitting or lateral position	Up to T10 and down to sacral area.
Hip surgery	0.5% heavy or plain bupivacaine 1.5–2 mls + diamorphine 300 mcg	Lateral position operative hip down if heavy bupivacaine, or uppermost if plain bupivacaine.	

Testing adequacy of anaesthesia

It's important to check that anaesthesia is adequate before proceeding with the operative procedure. This is most commonly done by using cold sensation as a surrogate for pain. Either 'cold spray' such as ethyl chloride can be used, or an ice cube, or failing that a cold glass ampoule taken from the fridge. It's important to test and document upper and lower limits of the block. One can also test absence of pain sensation using a needle or preferably by 'pinching' the skin (leaving lots of needle puncture marks doesn't look very nice!)

Common tip designs for spinal needles

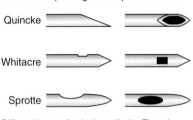

Quincke

Whitacre

Sprotte

Different types of spinal needle tip. There is evidence that not using a cutting-tip can reduce the incidence of post-procedure headache

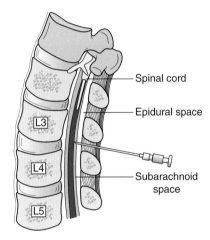

Spinal cord

Epidural space

Subarachnoid space

Spinal needle entering the subarachnoid space

OSCE checklist

- Assembles equipment correctly
- Positions patient appropriately
- Identifies and marks L4/5 interspace in midline
- Cleans skin
- Scrubs and dons appropriate sterile personal protective attire
- Applies sterile drape
- Raises a bleb of local anaesthetic under the skin
- Infiltrates local anaesthetic deeply
- Inserts spinal introducer needle
- Inserts spinal needle
- Removes the stylet
- Confirms correct position by observing drops of CSF
- Aspirates to re-confirm position
- Confirms correct drug prescribed and checks allergies
- Injects required drug
- Removes needle
- Presses on puncture site
- Washes hands
- Thanks patient
- Disposes of sharps and waste
- Documents procedure
- Provides postprocedure advice

36 Subcutaneous Injection

Rosemary Chester

Video Time | 1 min 43 s

Overview

It's five-o-clock and your tired little legs are approaching the end of a marathon post-take ward round comprising fifty patients no-less. Amongst your admissions, a lady presents with a long-standing history of malignancy and sudden onset of breathlessness associated with pleuritic chest pain and intermittent haemoptysis. On examination, you notice a tachycardia and, if you're lucky, auscultate a pleural rub. Alarmingly, you notice the oxygen saturations have been bobbing somewhere down around the patient's ankles. You strongly suspect a pulmonary embolism and prescribe a therapeutic dose of subcutaneous heparin which should be administered promptly, without delay. The CTPA you have swiftly organised merely confirms the diagnosis, but it's the anticoagulation therapy that ultimately treats it! Unfortunately, all of the nurses are busy in handover and your registrar asks you to kindly give the injection. It sounds simple as peas. Happy to proceed? Whilst the vast majority of injections in a ward setting are performed by nursing staff, it's important that you know how to perform the procedure too, should you find yourself in a similar scenario.

Subcutaneous injection is the giving of a drug into the fatty layer of soft tissue underneath the dermis and epidermis, and along with intravenous and intramuscular injections comprises one of three commonly used routes for administration of a multitude of drugs, used commonly in everyday practice in both medicine, surgery and out in the community. The subcutaneous plane is a relatively avascular, insulating layer of tissue, varying in depth obviously dependent on the BMI or 'body

How to Perform Clinical Procedures, First Edition. Matthew Stephenson, Joshua Shur and John Black.
© 2013 John Wiley & Sons, Ltd. Published 2013 by John Wiley & Sons, Ltd.

habitus' of said patient! There is little blood flow to the area compared to muscle for instance meaning the drug absorption rate is slow. Sometimes this can be anything up to 24 hours or longer depending on the drug in question. Typical medications administered subcutaneously are insulin, anticoagulant heparinoid products such as dalteparin or enoxaparin, and hormone injections (the initial two being far more commonplace and the latter is demonstrated in the accompanying video). Essentially, the technique for all of the above examples remains the same.

Indications	Contraindications	Complications
• Insulin injection • Subcutaneous heparin • Other drugs/ hormones	• Avoid repeated injection of the same site • Cellulitic/broken skin • Allergy to drug	• Bruising • Bleeding (mild to none) • Lipodystrophy • Fat necrosis (rare)

Procedure

Make sure you have the **correct patient**, for the **correct procedure**. Check for any **allergies**, and that you have confirmed the **indication;** excluded any **contraindications; explained** the procedure and taken **consent**. Now **wash your hands**!

Assemble all of your equipment on a sterile trolley away from the patient. You will need everything in the equipment textbox. It's important to understand which anatomical regions are appropriate for injection. The most common area for delivering a subcutaneous injection is the lower abdomen, but other acceptable sites include the upper arm, the lateral aspect of the thigh and the upper lateral quadrant of the derrière. Indeed, a change of injection site (if the therapy is regular, such as insulin) helps to prevent lipodystrophy (scarring and hardening of the tissues which can affect absorption rates). More importantly, it can be a source of chronic pain for the patient if they have to repeatedly inject into the same area.

You must check with the patient and their corresponding drug chart as to whether they have any **allergies**, and **always** be certain that your intended drug is not one they are sensitive to. This could

Equipment you need (on a sterile tray/trolley)

• Skin cleaning wipe
• Non-sterile gloves
• Orange (25G) needle
• Syringe filled with drug
• Cotton wool or sterile gauze
• Adhesive tape
• Sharps bin

lead to a cascade of mast-cell degranulation, general unpleasantness, and land you in sizeable amounts of trouble should you cause serious harm. Remember **you** are responsible as the prescriber.

Sometimes, the drug you are administering comes prepacked with a syringe, but in other cases, you may need to **prepare the drug**, drawing it up into a suitable syringe and/or possibly even diluting it with appropriate diluents – instructions for this will come with the drug.

Check the drug with a colleague – The five Rs offer a useful model before administration:

Right drug

Right dose

Right route

Right patient

Right date and time of administration

Finally, check the **expiry date** of the drug. Never give an out of date drug!

Wash your hands and **don your gloves**. It's a clean procedure, no sterile gloves required. **Inspect** for any obviously damaged areas of the overlying skin at the intended injection site, such as burns, areas of cellulitis, infection or eczema. Avoid previous injection sites where possible. **Clean the skin** with the alcohol preparation using ever increasing concentric circles outward from the site of intended puncture. **Allow it to dry** completely before proceeding.

Mount the needle on the syringe. Unsheath the needle and take the syringe in your dominant hand, holding it like a pencil. With the other hand, gently '**pinch**'

the skin between your thumb and index finger. **Warn the patient** of an imminent sharp scratch. Slowly **introduce the needle** at a 90° angle, or 45° angle in thin/muscular patients, advancing all the way to the hub (although the depth should be moderated again depending on the size of your patient). Release your pinch hold once fully introduced and **aspirate** on the syringe plunger to check for blood. In the absence of any aspirate, proceed to **inject the medication** at a steady rate over approximately 5–10 seconds, ensuring that the syringe is fully dispensed.

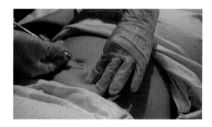

The fingers of the left hand are pinching up the skin and the needle is about to enter at about 45 degrees as this patient is relatively slim

As you **remove the needle** apply sterile gauze or cotton wool to the site and **apply moderate pressure**. This facilitates sealing of the puncture, prevents leakage and minimises the size of haematoma. You may notice a small amount of blood or fluid at the injection site – don't be alarmed! It's simply blood or a negligible amount of medication tracking along the injection site. You don't need to rub the injection site, this will just cause bruising. If necessary, stick the sterile gauze or cotton wool to the skin with a piece of adhesive tape. **Dispose of your sharps directly into** **the sharps bin** and any other **waste into the clinical waste bin** and **wash your hands**. Finally, remember to **sign, date and time** your prescription.

OSCE checklist

- Assembles equipment correctly
- Identifies injection site
- Checks drug chart
- Checks wrist band
- Confirms allergies with patient
- Checks drug expiry date
- Cleans area
- Pinches the skin
- Inserts needle at appropriate angle
- Administers drug correctly
- Disposes of sharp safely
- Signs drug chart
- Washes hands
- Thanks patient

37 Surgical Scrubbing

Shelly Griffiths

Video Time | 3 mins 29 s

Overview

Every doctor needs to know how to scrub, no matter what your future career intentions are! As well as in theatre itself, scrubbing and gowning is essential for more invasive procedures such as central venous lines. It is an easy procedure to perform, but an easy one to make frustrating mistakes in leaving you unsterile. Everyone has at some stage desterilised themselves while scrubbing or scrubbed – it's nothing to worry about, but you **must** always 'fess up and start again if this happens.

If you're called to theatre, you will be expected to know how to scrub. It's therefore advisable to have done it a few times whilst at medical school, and definitely before starting a surgical firm. Scrub nurses are the experts, so we advise finding a friendly one and asking them to run through the basics with you.

Procedure

As with all things, **preparation** is key. Make sure you have everything to hand before you start washing your hands.

The first step is to put on a **face mask**. Make sure it's comfortable and not in your eyes, as in many long procedures you will be unable to adjust it for several hours. Face masks can come with or without eye protection. If you're unsure if you need eye protection, always ask (or follow the example of the scrub nurse). As a basic rule, you will need eye protection for most orthopaedic procedures (certainly any using a drill or bone saw), vascular

Equipment you need

- Face mask (with or without eye protection)
- Sterile gown pack
- Correctly sized gloves
- Scrub sponge (opened)
- Assistant to help tie your gown

How to Perform Clinical Procedures, First Edition. Matthew Stephenson, Joshua Shur and John Black.
© 2013 John Wiley & Sons, Ltd. Published 2013 by John Wiley & Sons, Ltd.

procedures and anything messy (such as abscess drainage). Eye protection should also be worn when treating patients with blood-borne viruses. The face mask will contain a mouldable part over the nasal bridge which should be comfortably adjusted so that it fits snugly in place.

The **sterile gown pack** then needs to be opened. Open the packaging from the edges, pulling each corner of the pack apart to display the contents. Then open your **gloves** onto the pack. You will need to know your size, with most people being from a 5½ to 9. As a rough guide, most females take a 6–7 and males a 7–8. If available, a double glove pack can be used where necessary – this is normally again for orthopaedic cases or where a patient is a carrier of a blood-borne virus.

Before starting to scrub, **roll your sleeves** back to stop them getting in the way. **Turn on the taps** in the usual way: it's a good idea to spend a few seconds getting to a **comfortable water temperature**: too hot or too cold will result in an uncomfortable few minutes! **Rinse your hands** and **wash them** with scrub solution (see the following textbox), using your elbow to operate the dispenser. When you're washing your hands, make sure all surfaces are covered. If you are wearing a wedding band which you do not want to take off, move it up and down your finger whilst washing underneath its normal position. Then **rinse** your hands from the fingers towards the elbows, keeping the hands up so any dirty water runs away from your hands. Then begin your **scrub**,

There are two main types of scrub solution based on – **chlorhexidine** (pink) and **povidone-iodine** (brown). A number of studies have looked into which performs better, and the general consensus is that it's probably chlorhexidine, but that's still contentious and people use what they're comfortable with. Whichever you choose to use though, remember to use the same solution each time you scrub that day.

from hands to elbows. Make sure you scrub for long enough – 5 minutes for the first scrub of the day and 3 minutes for subsequent scrubs. For the specifics of how to actually wash your hands, that is, the different hand manoeuvres, check out Chapter 19 (Hand Hygiene, above).

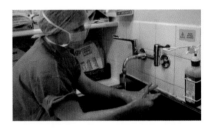

Note the sleeves are rolled up and the scrub has begun. Remember, if you must wear a wedding ring, wash underneath it

Use the **scrub sponge** for the first scrub of the day, **cleaning under your nails** with the brush and using the spongy side on skin. There is usually included a small instrument specifically cleaning under the fingernails which you can use. Some people find the scrub solution irritating when it's left on the skin, so make sure it's all thoroughly washed off. When you've finished, turn off the taps with your elbows and **keep your hands vertically upwards** to ensure dirty water runs away from them. **Dry your hands** using the sterile towels in the gown pack, again going from hands to elbows and using a separate towel for each arm.

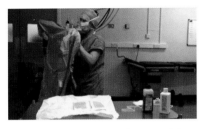

The gown is shaken open and you enter it from behind, as it were

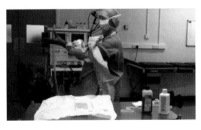

Note the overlap of gown cuff and glove

To put on the **gown** you'll need plenty of space so take a step back from the trolley. Hold either side and **shake it open** before putting your arms into the sleeves. An assistant will then normally tie up the back whilst you're putting on your **gloves**. The easiest way to put on the gloves is to place the glove against the palm of your hand with your thumb hooked into the cuff and then flip it over your fingers as demonstrated in the video. It will be more difficult if your hands are still wet, so make sure they are dried properly. To complete your scrub you just need to **tie the waist tie**. Take the cardboard tag and pass it to your assistant – complete a full 360° turn then pull the end of the tie out of the tag (which will stay in your assistant's hand) before tying it to the shorter tie attached to the gown.

Once you have scrubbed and gowned, remember that you are **sterile**! A basic rule to remember is not to touch **anything** which isn't blue. If you do accidentally de-sterilise yourself, firstly don't worry – we have all done it. You must however immediately leave the operating table and re-scrub.

OSCE checklist

- Places mask correctly
- Opens gown correctly
- Opens gloves onto sterile gown
- Rolls sleeves back
- Optimises water temperature
- Uses dispenser correctly
- Uses correct scrub technique
- Rinses hands correctly
- Scrubs hands for adequate time
- Closes taps with elbows
- Dries hands correctly
- Dons gown correctly
- Applies gloves
- Ties gown with assistant's help

38   Suturing

Video Time | 5 mins 58 s

Overview

Even the most committed anti-surgical abstract-thinking medic may be called upon to do a bit of suturing. Inpatients fall over and cut themselves. Drains need securing to the skin. Core biopsy wounds can bleed. And that's all before your A&E stint, where your suturing skills will be truly put to the test. So getting used to a needle holder and forceps (yes that's right, they're forceps not tweezers) is a basic skill for everyone to learn, even if you don't become super slick at it.

There are lots of different kinds of suture material, lots of different kinds of needle and lots of different ways of making a stitch and some of the common stitch types can be found in the accompanying figure. The interrupted suture is the most common, especially in A&E, as it lends itself to most kinds of wound.

Indications	Contraindications	Complications

• Wound closure
  ○ Iatrogenic
  ○ Traumatic
• Anchoring a drain, central line etc to the skin
	• Never close an infected wound – leave it open
	• A very deep wound – this may require open exploration in theatre for underlying tissue damage +/– deep layer closure
	• In children – consider using tissue adhesive glue (e.g. Dermabond) instead – it's far less painful!
		• Dehiscence (usually because your knot comes undone!)
		• Poor healing (usually because of one of the pitfalls discussed at the end of the chapter)
		• Infection
		• Bleeding
		• Poor cosmetic result

How to Perform Clinical Procedures, First Edition. Matthew Stephenson, Joshua Shur and John Black.
© 2013 John Wiley & Sons, Ltd. Published 2013 by John Wiley & Sons, Ltd.

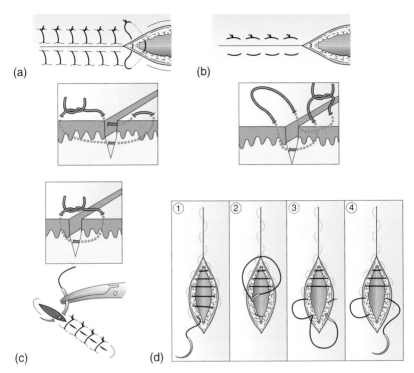

(a) Vertical mattress suture: often used when trying to close wound edges that are far apart, or that are deep; (b) horizontal mattress suture: used by some for personal preference; (c) interrupted suture: the basic, common garden suture that can be applied in many situations; (d) subcuticular: has the great advantages that it makes no holes in the skin therefore doesn't scar, and if absorbable suture is used, nothing needs to be removed

Procedure

So there are two contexts in which you will need to suture a wound, the first is when you've created the wound by removing a skin lesion for example, the second is if something else has created the wound – this you find in A&E. The only differences in terms of closure of the wound is that the latter is potentially dirty and should be cleaned thoroughly first, and sometimes the edges of the wounds need to be freshened up by trimming them if they look a bit ragged. For now, let's assume that this is a standard linear wound created on your patient's arm by a kitchen knife.

Make sure you have the **correct patient**, for the **correct procedure**. Check for any **allergies**, confirmed the **indication, explained the procedure** and that you've excluded any **contraindications** and taken **consent**. Now **wash your hands**!

Assemble all of your equipment on a sterile trolley away from the patient. You will need everything in the equipment textbox. This is a sterile procedure so you will need to wash your hands again thoroughly. When you have made the wound yourself by excising something, you should adopt full surgical sterile precautions, so this means formal scrubbing. In A&E, however, it's more commonly acceptable to just don **sterile gloves** and a non-sterile apron.

Clean the wound thoroughly with your hospital's preferred cleaning solution, for example Chlorhexidine or Betadine. If this looks like a fairly contaminated wound, and especially if you think there may be foreign material in there, **irrigate** it with copious amounts of normal saline using a syringe. **Never close a dirty wound**, consider leaving it open to heal by second intention, and this is often the best option if the wound was inflicted several hours ago and this is a delayed presentation. Just a reminder on this:

- Healing by *first intention*: The wound edges heal after being apposed together
- Healing by *second intention*: The wound edges are left apart and healing occurs from the base of the wound
- Healing by *delayed primary closure*: The wound edges are initially left to heal by second intention but are then closed formally later.

One other thing about dirty wounds, consider **tetanus prophylaxis**!

Create a **sterile field** around the wound with some sterile drapes, an aperture drape (which has a hole in the middle) is ideal. Inject some **local anaesthetic**, such as 1% lidocaine into the wound edges; see above Chapter 25: Local Anaesthetic Infiltration, for more on this.

For the purposes of closing the average wound, use something like a **2–0 Nylon suture** (a common trade name is Ethilon™, produced by Ethicon). It's non-absorbable and 'average' sized interms of suture width and it has a

---

Equipment you need (on a sterile tray/trolley)

- Sterile gloves +/– full sterile protective clothing (see above)
- Local anaesthetic (e.g., lidocaine 1%)
- Green needle (21G) to draw up local
- Blue needle (23G) to infiltrate local
- Syringe for the local
- Skin antiseptic
- A suture pack/kit, containing:
  - A needle holder
  - Pair of forceps
  - A pair of scissors
- At least one suture
- Sterile gauze
- Sterile drapes

cutting needle which works well for skin. **Mount your needle** in your needle holder and hold it with your dominant hand. You should be able to do this with your forceps and **never actually pick up the needle** with your fingers throughout the whole procedure. The needle should be mounted right **at the tip** of the needle holder, about **halfway round** the needle and **angled out slightly**. Some people prefer to mount the needle one third of the way round the needle and not angle it out. Try each style for yourself and see which you think works best.

Pick up the skin edge gently with your forceps. Gently means gently. Rough tissue handling results in tissue trauma and poor healing. Most people will use toothed forceps for this as these grab the skin in one tiny place rather than exerting pressure to a wide area of skin. **Insert the needle at a 90° angle** to the skin, approximately 5–10 mm away from the skin edge. **Supinate** your wrist so that you drive the needle through the tissue following the natural curve of the needle, and exit approx 5-10 mm in the subcutaneous tissue beneath the skin edge. Once you've driven it through the tissue as far as you can go, **use your forceps** to hold it momentarily, replace the needle holder a little closer to the needle point, let go with the forceps and pull the needle the rest of the way through the tissue. Ideally, when you remount the needle, you should remount it ready to

drive through the other skin edge. If not however, **pick up the needle** (which is now all the way through the first skin edge) with the forceps and remount the needle on the needle holder ready for the other skin edge.

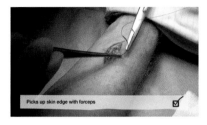

Picks up skin edge with forceps ☑

The first skin edge is held with the forceps and the needle is driven through at 90°

Pick up the other skin edge gently with your forceps and drive the needle into the subcutaneous tissue at the same depth from which your needle exited on the other side. It should enter at a **90° angle** to the subcutaneous tissue. Supinate your wrist like before and drive the needle through the subcutaneous tissue so it follows its natural curve and exits the skin at 90° to it. Again you may need to initially hold the needle with the forceps as it's coming out of the skin and then remount the needle a bit closer to the needle tip and pull it the rest of the way. Try not to hold the needle at the very tip though with the forceps or the needle holder as this can easily blunt it.

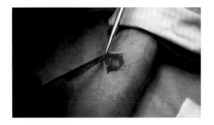

The needle is driven through the other skin edge

Now **tie the two ends** of suture together, either with a **hand tie** or **instrument tie**, whichever you prefer. This is far better explained with a video than in text, so check this out on the DVD. It's important to remember that you only want the two edges to be **gently apposed** for them to heal, you don't need to squeeze them together with an over tight knot which just risks rendering them ischaemic. **Cut the suture** to about 1 cm length. Too short and it's more difficult to get hold of when it comes to removing it, too long and the ends irritate the adjacent skin. Make sure that the knots all land up resting at the sides, that is, not over the

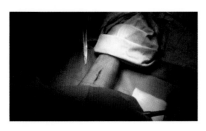

The suture is tied

wound itself which may disturb healing. It looks prettier if they all end up the same side, and the district nurse is less likely to privately cuss your handiwork when she takes them out.

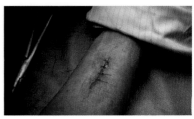

The finished row of sutures

Repeat the process and put in as many sutures as you need to bring the wound edges together, leaving 5–10 mm space between them. You may be able to get several stitches out of one suture if you're sparing with it. Finally **clean the skin** again with sterile water or normal saline, washing off any antiseptic solution and blood. Apply a **sterile dressing** over the wound.

If you're using non-absorbable sutures you need to leave **postprocedure instructions** for when they need to come out so that the patient's practice nurse can do this and you also need to give some wound care advice. The average time for asking for sutures to be removed is 7 days; however, if the skin edges have had to be pulled together, such as if a large skin lesion was removed, they may be under a little tension, so you may opt to leave them in even for up to 2 weeks. In contrast, for a small wound that's been sutured on the face, it's better to remove the sutures as early as 3–5 days. This is because sutures, especially if they're thick, can cause scarring too and furthermore wounds on the face tend to heal very quickly because of the excellent blood supply. So on the face, use a narrower suture and take it out sooner.

Common pitfalls

The correct way for the skin to be closed is for the edges to be simply apposed against each other, as shown in the correct method for suturing in the accompanying figure. A common problem as mentioned above is for the edges to be pulled too tight which can render them ischaemic, or for one edge to ride up over the other and overlap or for the two edges to invert. If anything, the edges should slightly evert, and definitely not invert. Two layers of epidermis drawn together in apposition won't heal!

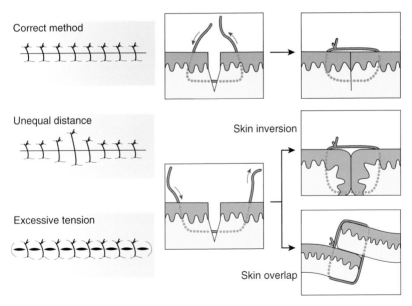

Correct method

Unequal distance

Excessive tension

Skin inversion

Skin overlap

The most common errors in wound closure

OSCE checklist

- Assembles equipment correctly
- Administers local anaesthetic
- Mounts needle correctly
- Handles equipment appropriately
- Picks up skin edge with forceps
- Drives needle through skin edge at 90°
- Uses forceps to help passage of needle
- Drives needle through other skin edge at equal depth
- Performs secure knot
- Snugs the knot down over the skin not the wound
- Cuts suture to appropriate length
- Inserts following sutures at appropriate distances
- Completes skin closure
- Cleans skin and applies dressing
- Washes hands
- Thanks patient
- Disposes of sharps and waste
- Documents procedure
- Provides postprocedure advice

39 Urinalysis

Aisling Hilary

Video Time | 4 mins 24 s

Overview

All too frequently, the diagnostic potential of a good old urine sample is overlooked. Whoever invented the urine dipstick and pregnancy test deserves a gold medal and crowned king, or queen, of the cost-effective bedside procedures. Dipping a patient's urine can be an extremely quick and rewarding test that often gives you a wealth of insight. It's quick, it's cheap, it's easy to do, and used in the correct context (along with a thorough history and examination) has a high sensitivity despite its relative simplicity. In light of the above, it's important to have a grasp on how to perform a urine dip, the potential diagnoses and also have a handle on how to interpret the results.

It's important to highlight the urinary pregnancy test too. **Every female patient presenting with abdominal pain, of child bearing age should have a urinary pregnancy test**. There really is no excuse not to do this, as it may be the difference, quite literally between life and death by diagnosing for instance, an ectopic pregnancy. It goes without saying that women of child bearing age should also have a pregnancy test if it's possible that their symptoms could be related to pregnancy, or if the management might be affected by one (e.g. if the patient may need x-rays).

A urinary pregnancy test can, of course give a false positive or false negative result, and the result should therefore be interpreted with caution. Urinary pregnancy tests are considered more reliable after 6 weeks gestation. So with the vast majority of ectopics presenting after 6 weeks gestation (when a urinary pregnancy test is more reliable), it's an excellent diagnostic tool of exclusion. If suspicion is high following a careful history, this should be backed up with

How to Perform Clinical Procedures, First Edition. Matthew Stephenson, Joshua Shur and John Black.
© 2013 John Wiley & Sons, Ltd. Published 2013 by John Wiley & Sons, Ltd.

serum beta-HCG and progesterone levels (which invariably surpasses the expected levels estimated for 'weeks of gestation' in the case of an ectopic). So please… always, **always** do it.

Indications	Contraindications	Complications
• Fever (as part of septic screen) • Dysuria • Polyuria • Urinary frequency • Confusion (in the elderly) • Urinary incontinence (elderly and children) • Abdominal pain • Haematuria • Late menses • Suspicion of pregnancy	• Avoid old urine samples/leg bags/collection devices • Pregnancy test: Interpret with caution up to 6 weeks' gestation.	• False positive/ negative pregnancy test

Procedure

Urine collection

If the patient is mobile, not systemically compromised and producing urine, provide them with a sterile bowl and kindly request they relieve themselves into it.

If the indication for urinalysis is to look for infection then you wish to sample the urine in the bladder, not the urine that's trickled over the surface of a dirty glans penis or unwashed labia. So make sure you instruct a man to pull back the foreskin and wash the penis before weeing, and for a woman to wash around the urethral meatus and part the labia during micturition. In both cases, the first bit of urine out should be discarded, that is, wee it straight out into the toilet, this

volume effectively washes out the urethra. You are looking for a **midstream urine sample** (**MSU**).

If your patient requires a urinary catheter, then you should aim to obtain a 'clean catch' at the point of catheterisation. This means, once you've inserted the catheter, allow the first few drops to drip away and then collect your sample into a sterile white topped pot. This is not an MSU, this is a **Catheter Specimen of Urine** (**CSU**).

Finally, if the patient has an indwelling catheter, you will need to syringe out a sample of fresh urine, as opposed to a sample of urine that has been festering for the last 12 hours in a leg bag. Stagnant urine is likely to contain bacteria, making your urine dipstick glow. You can do this by taking a green (21G) needle and syringe to the bedside. You will find along the length of the catheter tubing, a port with a rubber diaphragm. You can clean this with some sterile wipes and insert the needle through it and aspirate directly from the catheter tube. Again, this is a CSU obviously.

For completeness, you can also take a suprapubic sample, however we will not discuss this method any further.

When sending your sample to the lab, make sure you document what type of specimen has been collected as this is important to direct the microbiologist.

Equipment you need (on a sterile tray/trolley)

- Sterile urinary bowl/pot
- Gloves
- White top urine bottle
- Red top urine bottle
- Urine dip tests strips
- Urine dip test developing chart (on the bottle)
- Urine sample
- Pregnancy test kit (strip and pipette)
- Sample request form

Urinalysis

Once the sample has been obtained you are ready to test it. The urine dipstick comes as a **universal standard**, and tests for the following: glucose, ketones, specific gravity (how concentrated the urine is), blood, protein, nitrites and leucocytes. It will also measure a pH. The strips are extremely sensitive not only to moisture, but also light. Therefore you will find them readily available on most wards, normally in the sluice areas in a blacked out, lidded container.

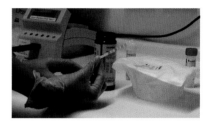

The equipment needed

For ease, **decant the urine** from the large collection bowl into a **white-top** bottle. These are also found on the wards, with a neighbouring **red-top** urine sample bottle. It's worth noting that the red top contains a **boric acid medium**, which fixes the urine sample and its contents, preparing it for MC + S. The white top bottle contains no such medium. Never dipstick urine from a red top – it will of course always skew the pH and other test results.

Wash your hands and put on some **gloves** – non sterile gloves are fine for this procedure. Unscrew the lid from the urine sample carefully, avoiding spillage, holding it in your non-dominant hand. Take a suitable dipstick test strip in your dominant hand and fully **submerge the strip** into your urine pot for approximately 5 seconds, **withdrawing the stick** and **carefully placing the urine sample down**.

Still holding the test strip in your dominant hand, pick up the test strip container and **begin timing**. The glucose is the first test to develop after approximately 30 seconds. Ketones are next, at around 40 seconds followed by specific gravity, blood, protein, nitrites and finally leucocytes at approximately 2 minutes. The bottle containing the dipsticks has a key for these. Make a note of any positive findings, using the colour chart on the test strip bottle to identify the abundance of various substances being tested for. Remember, you should only assess the dipstick after the time is up and not reassess it 2 minutes later or similar, the result will not be accurate. You may find an **automated machine** in your hospital (as in the video) which does all the analysis for you and prints out a result almost instantaneously.

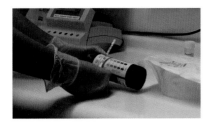

The urine dipstick has been dipped in the urine and is held against the bottle with the colour code on it

If the urine dipstick is positive for infection (i.e. protein and nitrites/leucocytes +/− blood), then the urine should be sent for **microscopy, culture and sensitivity** (MC + S). Carefully decant the urine into a **red top bottle**, as this is required for further laboratory testing, giving you an idea of the causative organism and its relevant antibiotic sensitivities. Carefully **label** the sample with the patient's details and complete the necessary request form with matching patient details and sample type.

Pregnancy tests all too often are accompanied by an air of uncertainty and confusion, simply due to the wealth of variation currently available on today's market. However, the test strip you will find in hospitals is relatively standardised in attempts for uniformity and to render it user friendly.

The test usually takes the form of a pre-packed entity, consisting of the test strip, a small pipette and a really rather convoluted set of instructions. The test strip will have a 'well' at one end and a 'window' at the other. Wearing gloves (remember you are handling a bodily fluid after all) carefully **fill the pipette** with the patient's urine to be tested, and **dispatch 3 drops** (this may vary according to manufacturer, so remember to read the instructions carefully if you are not familiar with the testing kit) **into the well of the test strip**. You then have to **wait**, usually 3 minutes.

At the viewing window, you will see one of two things: one line normally indicates that the urine tested does **not** contain beta HCG, thus is a negative pregnancy test. Two lines normally confirms the presence of beta HCG, thus confirming a positive urinary pregnancy test. Do remember to wait for the full three minutes, as in small concentrations (i.e. earlier pregnancy) the test can take longer to develop. The positive line may be very faint or ambiguous – in this case you should send the patient's blood for a serum level, and there is no harm in repeating the pregnancy test for replication/validation of the result.

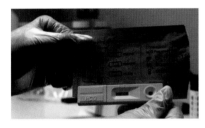

A pregnancy test with accompanying instructions

Once you have completed your necessary testing, remember to carefully **document** your finding with a dated, timed and signed entry in the patients clinical notes. Make a note of the pregnancy test batch number and record this alongside any findings.

Act on any findings as soon as possible. If you're unsure, use your peers. The nurses on the ward will almost certainly be more experienced at these simple, yet valuable bedside tests, and should be of great assistance. Make use of their expertise.

Finally, remember to throw the remnants of your sample into the sluice and **dispose of it correctly**. Throw away your used kits and tidy up any spilt urine. **Wash your hands**, and remember to drop any samples off to the lab for prompt analysis.

OSCE checklist

- Assembles equipment correctly
- Checks date and integrity of urine dipstick
- Submerges the stick appropriately
- Interprets results accurately in a timely manner
- Understands electronic analysis
- Cleans equipment
- Obtains results and adds to patient's notes
- Transfers urine to red top bottle
- Labels bottle and completes request form appropriately
- Dispenses 3 drops into well of pregnancy strip
- Adheres to sample time
- Interprets results accurately
- Understands when repeat indicated / further investigation required
- Disposes of biological waste safely
- Washes hands
- Thanks patient

40 Urinary Catheter – Female

Video Time | 4 mins 16 s

Overview

Probably more so than any other procedure over the last decade or so, female catheterisations have almost completely been usurped by nurses. The reason is obvious, most nurses are of the lady variety, so it only seems natural that they would undertake such an intimate procedure. However, the time will come one day when you're on the ward faced with a critically unwell female patient needing urine output monitoring, or the less common female urinary retention – and all the nurses are male, or the one lady nurse is on her break, or some similar farce. You will particularly be called upon to catheterise a female patient in theatre – this task falls to the most junior medical member of staff. However in reality, training and experience rather than gender should be the main criterion when performing this procedure.

The good news is it's really, really easy. Easier than a male catheterisation. However, even for the most perineally self-aware lady doctor or the most adventurous Casanova of a male doctor, the lady-parts can on occasion be somewhat perplexing (particularly in the elderly or obese)– but it all becomes clear with one basic manoeuvre, so read on.

Below are the general indications, contraindications and complications. It is worth mentioning that urinary incontinence and immobility are **not** usually acceptable indications. Good nursing and medical care, with less invasive interventions (such as absorbant pads) are often enough. Catheterisation should always be a last resort in such cases and where catheterisation is required long term for these indications, this is best achieved with a suprapubic catheter.

How to Perform Clinical Procedures, First Edition. Matthew Stephenson, Joshua Shur and John Black.
© 2013 John Wiley & Sons, Ltd. Published 2013 by John Wiley & Sons, Ltd.

Indications	Contraindications	Complications
• Monitoring of renal function • Intravesical chemotherapy • Urinary retention (uncommon) • Rarely, urinary incontinence or very immobile patients (see above)	• Suspected urethral trauma • Previous traumatic catheterisation	• Urinary infection • Blockage • Urethral irritation/bleeding

Complications such as urosepsis and trauma do occur, and can be serious, even fatal. For that reason it's really important to consider carefully the clinical need for catherisation. If you can get away without it, try not to place one. Nowadays most trusts will have a catheter care bundle which are strictly audited. Nursing staff will need to sign daily that they have reviewed the indication for catheterisation. As soon as it's no longer needed, take it out.

This is a standard 2-way catheter. There are also **3-way catheters** which have an extra port and lumen which is used for **irrigation** of the bladder. This comes in handy for example, if the patient has haematuria, as stagnant bloody urine will tend to clot, but by constantly irrigating the bladder, you reduce the risk of 'clot retention'.

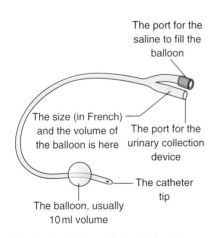

The port for the saline to fill the balloon

The size (in French) and the volume of the balloon is here

The port for the urinary collection device

The catheter tip

The balloon, usually 10 ml volume

The standard urinary catheter with 2 ports

Procedure

Make sure you have the **correct patient**, for the **correct procedure**. Check for any **allergies**, and that you have confirmed the **indication;** excluded any **contraindications; explained** the procedure and taken **consent**. Now **wash your hands**!

Assemble all of your equipment on a trolley away from the patient and before you have exposed them. You will need everything in the equipment textbox. Open the prepackaged sterile equipment in the usual aseptic manner onto your sterile field contained within the catheter pack. Take care not to contaminate the field. As always with such an invasive procedure, a completely **aseptic technique is mandatory**. In some trusts, a **prophylactic dose of antibiotics** like 80 mg gentamycin IM, is given to all patients just before the catheterisation, and is certainly a good idea for immunocompromised patients. Check your trust's guidelines.

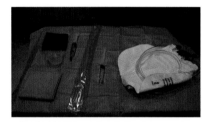

The equipment laid out on a sterile trolley

Equipment you need (on a sterile tray/trolley)

- Sterile catheter pack containing:
  - Sterile gloves
  - Sterile field
  - Waste bag
  - A gallipot
  - Cotton wool balls or similar
  - Gauze swabs
  - Plastic tray
- A second pair of sterile gloves (depending on your technique)
- Lubricating anaesthetising gel (e.g. Instillagel)
- Cleaning solution
- Sterile water in a syringe (usually 10 ml) to inflate balloon
- The urinary catheter (usually start with 14 or 16 F)
- The urine collection bag or urometer
- Apron

Looking at a standard urinary catheter, you'll notice there are **two ports** on the end – one communicates with the wider lumen that runs the length of the catheter, **urine** will come out here. The other port communicates with a narrower lumen which connects with an **inflatable balloon** at the business end of the catheter, which will hold the catheter in the bladder. It's sensible to remove the packaging from this end of the catheter to **connect the urine drainage bag** to the urine port, **and the sterile water filled syringe** to the other port, right now before you even approach the patient. This will save you from doing it later when you are draining urine. Some people however prefer to connect these once they have placed the catheter. However, leave the rest of the catheter wrapping in place for now.

Once you have your equipment ready, stand to the patient's right and **uncover the patient** so that the perineum is exposed and ask the patient to raise their knees with the heels together, and then let their **legs gently flop outwards**. This can be difficult for patients with arthritic hips or knees. It's at this stage that you might look between the legs and wonder where on earth you're going to find the right orifice. This is simply because the labia majora can sometimes become very floppy and lax and cover over the external urethral meatus and vaginal orifice. So, use your left hand (assuming you're right handed, but if you're an incontrovertible lefty, you may want to switch sides here), usually the 2nd and 3rd fingers, to **lift up the labia majora to reveal the anatomy**. In some patients, especially elderly and obese patients, the external urethral meatus may not be immediately apparent as additional skin folds or the labia minora can trick you into thinking there is a meatus. As long as you lift up well enough with your left hand – and this is the **key manoeuvre** – it will become very obvious. The **external urethral meatus is the most anterior orifice**.

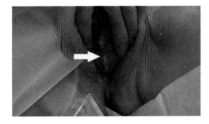

The arrow is pointing to the external urethral meatus

Next **clean the area**. Your left hand remains lifting up the labia majora, and use the right hand to **wipe the perineum**, front to back, over the external urethral meatus. **Repeat** this two or three times. The next important concept to grasp is that your left hand is now dirty – it must not touch any of the important bits of sterile equipment – its job is essentially to lift the labia. The right hand does all the rest of the work. This is the so-called '**one handed**

technique'. In reality, you do still use the left hand occasionally to help peel back the catheter wrapping for instance, but it only touches things that are not going to come in contact with the patient.

Open up the **sterile drape** between the patient's legs and move the rest of your equipment from the sterile trolley to the drape. Some people prefer to use an aperture drape for this procedure. **Insert some lubricating anaesthetising gel** (e.g. Instillagel) into the external urethral meatus. You will need less of course than a male as the urethra is much shorter. Your trust may have a specific guideline on how much to use, or even a smaller volume 'female' syringe – so it's best to check first.

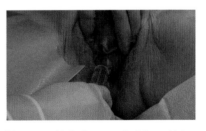

Inject some lubricating anaesthetizing gel into the external urethral meatus

Peel the wrapping off just the tip of the catheter (your dirty left hand can help because this wrapper isn't going to enter the bladder or touch the catheter again). **Pass the catheter into the bladder**, and peel a bit more of the wrapper off the catheter. Repeat this alternating movement until the catheter is about 8 cm inside. This is enough for the tip and the balloon to be comfortably inside, yet not so far that the catheter might have passed through the bladder and up a ureter (i.e. you don't need to insert it to the hilt like in a male)! Once you're in by 8 cm, **check that urine is flowing back** through the catheter. That is the most important thing to look for, as this confirms you are in the bladder. **Inflate the balloon** fully by injecting the sterile water filled syringe. It's much easier if this and the urine collection device has been already attached – doing it now with one hand is difficult. It also means you don't have to play the game of 'race the urine' where you're rapidly trying to fit the urine collection bag on whilst watching the urine stream down the catheter and out over your hand.

Gently withdraw the catheter until you meet resistance – this is just the

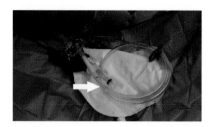
Urinary flashback into the catheter

balloon abutting against the internal urethral meatus and confirms the catheter is in place and that the balloon has filled (and hasn't popped). **Remove the rest of the wrapping** from the catheter and as soon as possible, **cover the patient back up**.

Finally **clean up** – make sure you wipe off any excess lubricating gel or spilt urine. Dispose of your gloves and equipment in a clinical waste bin.

In most hospital trusts it is now policy to **take the sticker** from the catheter wrapper and put it in the notes alongside where you will next **document the procedure** you have performed. Make sure to record what size and type of catheter was placed, whether it was an easy or difficult catheterisation, the amount of water used to inflate the balloon, colour of urine and any debris or blood present and if any urine samples have been sent. Also document the residual volume.

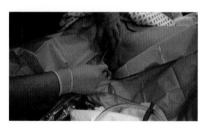
The catheter just entering the urethra, note the hands don't touch the catheter itself

OSCE checklist

- Assembles equipment correctly
- Connects drainage bag and syringe to catheter
- Positions patient correctly
- Uses 'one hand' technique
- Cleans around external urethral meatus
- Creates a sterile field
- Identifies external urethral meatus
- Injects lubricating gel into meatus
- Peels back wrapping from catheter tip
- Inserts catheter into meatus
- Checks for urinary 'flashback'
- Advances catheter without touching it
- Inflates balloon
- Gently withdraws catheter until resistance is met
- Removes rest of wrapping
- Cleans area and disposes of waste
- Re-covers patient promptly
- Washes hands
- Thanks patient
- Documents procedure
- Provides postprocedure advice

41 Urinary Catheter – Male

Video Time | 3 mins 34 s

Overview

Urethral catheterisation is the insertion of a catheter through the external urethral meatus and into the bladder to allow free flow of urine. It's a very common procedure and although it's performed strictly as an aseptic technique, catheterisation is permitted to be performed as a ward-based procedure.

There's no doubt as a junior doctor you will receive a bleep requesting your expertise to perform the task of inserting a male urethral catheter. Due to sensitivity issues, you may have had little to no experience at medical school. In some trusts there is an unwritten rule that men should only perform male catheters, and females should only perform female catheters. In truth however, anyone who is properly trained should be able to perform this procedure, regardless of gender. Remember, for many patients this is often a highly invasive and embarrassing procedure. Demonstrate an absolute air of sensitivity throughout, and you will make the whole process a little more bearable for your patient.

Now one must always question the reason for inserting a foreign object into a penis. Despite the most generous of lubrication, catheterisation remains potentially traumatic to the epithelial lining of the urethral tract, and the potential for inadvertent introduction of infection remains significant. It's important to have an absolute indication and weigh up the risk versus the benefit, whilst at the same time considering potential contraindications. A common indication is that the patient has gone into urinary retention and is unable to pass urine, which is extremely unpleasant and painful. Imagine the discomfort associated with that seemingly endless coach journey (we've all been there), where you are just **desperate** to go, and

How to Perform Clinical Procedures, First Edition. Matthew Stephenson, Joshua Shur and John Black.
© 2013 John Wiley & Sons, Ltd. Published 2013 by John Wiley & Sons, Ltd.

multiply by a million. You can become the patient's best friend forever if you promptly relieve them by inserting a catheter. Other indications include: accurate fluid management in a septic patient, pre/postoperative care and very rarely in the management of urinary incontinence coupled with immobility however good nursing and medical care should make this extremely rare.

A dazzling array of catheters are available in terms of design and appearance, and again this usually boils down to manufacturer and branding. Simplified, catheters vary in size, both in girth and length, the material they are made of (PTFE or acrylic), and the number of ports (dual port or three-way). Catheter girth is measured in French Charriere's units and choice of catheter size needs to be individualised to the patient. Current best practice is to insert a 16 F for a male and a 12 F for a female, sizes which are judged as the smallest catheter that will allow for free flow of urine without the urine bypassing the catheter. The catheter will also come with a 10 ml syringe of sterile water to inflate the catheter balloon once in the bladder. Bear in mind that whilst in the past there were two different catheter lengths, one for females and one for males, this is no longer recommended and all patients should be catheterised with a 'male' catheter (see Chapter 40: Urinary Catheter – Female).

You may be more familiar with the yellow catheters which are often made out of polyvinyl chloride or Teflon coated with a latex core. These are both short-term catheters which should not remain in situ for longer than 7 days or 28 days respectively. There are also long-term catheters which are made out of silicone, often clear or blue in colour to differentiate, and may remain in situ for up to 12 weeks.

For more about the urinary catheter itself, see Chapter 40: Urinary Catheter – Female.

Indications	Contraindications	Complications
• Urinary retention • Monitoring of fluid balance • Intravesical chemotherapy • Rarely, urinary incontinence or very immobile patients (see above)	• Suspected urethral trauma • Previous traumatic catheterisation • Urethral stricture • Bifid urethra	• Urinary infection • Blockage • Urethral irritation/bleeding

Procedure

Make sure you have the **correct patient**, for the **correct procedure**. Check for any **allergies**, and that you have confirmed the **indication;** excluded any **contraindications; explained** the procedure and taken **consent**. Now **wash your hands**!

Assemble all of your equipment on a trolley away from the patient and before you have exposed them. You will need everything in the equipment textbox. Open the prepackaged sterile equipment in the usual aseptic manner onto your sterile field contained within the catheter pack. In order to optimise your technique, you may consider connecting the sterile water (used to inflate the balloon) to the balloon port, and connect the other port to the collection bag before you start to avoid urine spillage. This will make you look slicker, but it remains optional (it is shown in the female catheter video but not in the male catheter video).

As always with such an invasive procedure, a completely **aseptic technique is mandatory**. In some trusts, a **prophylactic dose of antibiotics** like 80 mg gentamycin IM, is given to all patients just before the catheterisation, and is certainly a good idea for immuno-compromised patients. Check your trust's guidelines.

Position the patient supine. Elevate the bed to ensure you are in a comfortable position. **Maintain privacy and dignity** by ensuring he is not unnecessarily exposed. However, now is the time to **uncover the genitals** and **retract the foreskin** (if they have one).

Equipment you need (on a sterile tray/trolley)

- Sterile catheter pack containing:
  - Sterile gloves
  - Sterile field
  - Waste bag
  - A gallipot
  - Cotton wool balls or similar
  - Gauze swabs
  - Plastic tray
- A second pair of sterile gloves (depending on your technique)
- Lubricating anaesthetising gel (e.g. Instillagel)
- Cleaning solution
- Sterile water in a syringe (usually 10 ml) to inflate balloon
- The urinary catheter (usually start with 14 or 16 F)
- The urine collection bag or urometer
- Apron

Put on a disposable apron and **don your sterile gloves**. The general etiquette is to approach the patient from the right hand side. Proceed to **make a hole in the sterile field** and place this around the penis. Use the sterile gauze or cotton wool balls dipped in cleansing solution (in accordance with trust policy) to **clean the glans penis**. Start at the meatus and wipe away concentrically, removing any smegma or detritus. A useful tip is to use one of the pieces of gauze as a sling around the penis during this procedure, which further minimises the risk of penis-hand contact.

Use the **lubricating anaesthetic gel**, such as Instillagel by initially applying a small amount around the urethral opening and then insert the tip into the urethra. Inject plenty of the gel into the urethra, leaving some to lubricate the tip of the catheter before insertion. This is most important. The meatal orifice should not invert as you pass the catheter, so **lube up real good**. If necessary, use a second syringe. Ensure you hold the penis perpendicular and apply a small amount of pressure at the tip of the glans to ensure the gel doesn't simply flow back out. Patience is a virtue at this point and you should **wait for 3–5 minutes** to allow for the anaesthetic to take effect. This can seem like the longest 3–5 minutes of your life, so perhaps have a spiel of small talk prepared to fill awkward silences.

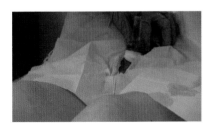

The penis is held at 90 degrees and lubricating anaesthetising gel is injected

Discard the first pair of gloves and **don the second pair**. Tear off the end of the catheter wrapping to **expose the tip**. **Hold the penis at** **90°** with a swab in your left hand. The next important concept to grasp is that your left hand is now dirty – it must not touch any of the important bits of sterile equipment – its job is essentially to hold the penis. The right hand does all the rest of the work. This is the so-called '**one-handed technique**'. In reality, you do still use the left hand occasionally to help peel back the catheter wrapping for instance, but it only touches things that are not going to come in contact with the patient.

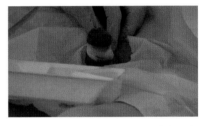

The catheter enters the urethra, note the hands never actually touch the catheter

Using your right hand **insert the tip of the catheter** into the penis. **Advance the catheter** all the way until the bifurcation is reached. To do this you need to **avoid touching the catheter itself**, you only touch the wrapping. This takes a bit of practice as you need to gradually peel a bit of the wrapping off, advance the catheter a little, peel back more wrapping, advance the catheter a bit more etc. Urine should begin to flow once the catheter is fully in. It may take a few seconds or more if you've used lots of gel – be patient, if you're sure you're in the bladder, it will come eventually.

If there is resistance on insertion you may ask the patient to cough which may reduce spasm of the external sphincter. Additionally you may ask the patient to thrust their pelvis forwards to change the angle of insertion especially if they have an enlarged prostate. However **never push hard** if you encounter resistance. Experience will tell you how much is safe pressure. Serious damage can be done with a urinary catheter by creating blind passages. With the catheter advanced to the bifurcation and urine flowing out, **inflate the balloon** with the 10 mls of sterile water. Ensure to apply continual pressure to the syringe until you have disconnected from the balloon port. Failure to do so will result in back-flow of the sterile water re-entering the syringe and an underinflated balloon: the catheter will fall out. **Withdraw the catheter** until resistance is felt as the balloon abuts the internal urethral meatus. **Attach a catheter bag**, **clean the patient** and always remember to **reposition the foreskin**. **This is most important to avoid paraphimosis**. Dispose of any **clinical waste**. Take a **sample of urine** for urinalysis and culture if appropriate and measure the residual volume. If the patient is mobile

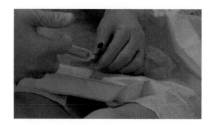

The balloon is inflated via the other port once urinary flashback is observed and the catheter is all the way up to the hilt.

you can use a leg back to keep them ambulant. Use the purposely-designed leg straps to immobilise the tubing and prevent tugging on the catheter which is very painful.

You must **document** everything you've done in the notes including the type and size of catheter used, amount of sterile water inserted into the balloon, findings from the urinalysis (if performed) and residual volume in the notes. Also comment on the physical appearance of the urine and presence of any frank haematuria or clots. Ensure the **batch number stickers** on the external aspect of the catheter packaging are completed (it's very self explanatory) and placed in the notes. If the reason for catheterisation was due to retention you should also perform a **digital rectal examination** to assess the prostate. Remember to document all of the above along with relevant examination findings.

OSCE checklist

- Assembles equipment correctly
- Dons apron
- Exposes patient
- Dons gloves
- Places sterile field
- Retracts foreskin
- Places sling around penis
- Cleans glans
- Administers instillagel
- Opens catheter pack
- Lubricates catheter tip
- Inserts catheter into penis
- Uses aseptic non touch technique to insert catheter
- Advances catheter all the way to the hilt
- Inflates balloon with sterile water
- Asks patient about pain
- Withdraws catheter until resistance is met
- Attaches catheter bag
- Replaces foreskin
- Removes sterile field
- Ensures the patient is clean and comfortable
- Documents the procedure including residual volume
- Sends a specimen for M,C + S if required or completes a urine dip
- Washes hands
- Thanks patient

42 Venepuncture

Video Time | 3 mins 39 s

Overview

'Taking blood' is one of the *most* common invasive procedures – you and your nursing colleagues will have to do it all the time. Thankfully for the junior doctors of today, taking blood is now performed by all sorts of clinical practitioners including nurses, phlebotomists, midwives and health care assistants. This undoubtedly has made our lives easier. However, it's a real risk that you can deskill from this very basic task. By 3 months into your F1 year, you should be able to bleed anyone or anything at any time of the day or night with one arm tied behind your back, blindfolded. If you always let the phlebotomists or the nurses do it, you're really missing out on gaining a vital clinical skill.

Blood tests form one of the pillars of basic clinical investigation and as such all patients admitted to hospital will have them taken in one form or another. If you are on a surgical firm then you will have to make sure that your patients have been group and screened and had haemoglobin and clotting checked before theatre for instance. At a crash call you will have to send off bloods as an emergency to check for biochemical or haematological causes for the patient's demise. It's difficult to envisage any post take ward round taking place without reviewing a patient's blood results.

Because it's so common you are probably reading this and thinking *everyone knows how to take blood – why did you need to write a chapter about it?* The authors sympathise but there are important reasons to labour on about it.

Firstly because it's so common it should *not* be done badly, and believe us, it is often still done very badly. This is important as no invasive procedure is without risks or complications. Secondly some patients have blood taken very frequently. Doing it

How to Perform Clinical Procedures, First Edition. Matthew Stephenson, Joshua Shur and John Black.

well minimises pain, can improve patient compliance and is best practice. Thirdly people DO needle stick themselves performing venepuncture- a few extra hints and tips could actually help reduce this. Fourthly an aseptic technique is often ignored in practice but is essential to reduce the risk of introducing a bacteraemia.

Anatomy

Before we start with the basic anatomy we should point out that you can pretty much take blood from any decent vein – and sometimes, if nothing else is available these might be found on the feet or with babies on their scalp for instance.

We will focus on the most common places however and these are found on the upper limb. The best veins are usually found over the forearm or over the back of the hand. In the antecubital fossa this will most likely be the median cubital vein and on the back of the hand the cephalic vein (laterally) and the basilic vein (medially). The cephalic vein as it passes over the head of the radius is a great site and accordingly is known as the houseman's vein. Beware also, that for patients with chronic kidney disease who are on dialysis or who may need it in the future – their more proximal

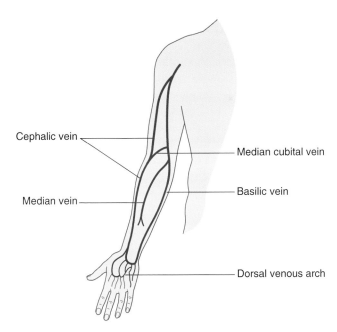

A schematic of the venous anatomy of the upper limb

veins must be preserved in case they need a fistula. This means only taking blood from the backs of the hands.

It is worth remembering that the brachial artery along with the median nerve is lurking just medial to the insertion of the biceps tendon.

The different options for taking blood

There are many ways to take blood and each has its advocates who will fiercely defend it and criticise the others. Before we go into the details let's just recap the main ways you can take blood:

1 *Needle and syringe*. The traditional method. Pros: Pretty much any ward carries a needle and syringe. Cheap. Cons: You have to then separately get the blood into the blood bottles increasing the risk of needle-stick and risk of the blood haemolysing. This method is disapproved of nowadays by most, mainly because of the needle stick injury risk and we would therefore not recommend it.

2 *Vacutainer with winged needle ('butterfly')*. Pros: Most people find the butterfly easier to use. You don't need to transfer the blood into the bottles afterwards. Cons: Some people don't like the vacutainer.

3 *Vacutainer with needle*. Pros: Low risk of needle-stick (you don't need to fill the bottles afterwards). Cons: Some of these sets don't give a 'flashback' making it more difficult to use as you can't be sure you're in the vein.

4 *Butterfly and syringe*. This is many people's favourite. Pros: Easy to see when you are in a vein. Can draw off as much blood as you need. Cons: More expensive, still have to transfer the blood into the bottles, risking a needlestick injury.

The Vacutainer method with a needle has become *the* preferred method in many trusts and for that reason we will explain how to use it-in fact method two and three are the only ones that are recommended these days.

The Vacutainer system is the trade name for a collection method that has become increasingly popular. Essentially there is a collection device which you can push blood bottles into. This means that the blood bottles are filled at the bedside and you do not have to fill them later. This reduces the chance of a sampling error and also reduces the chance of a needle-stick as you do not need use a needle to fill the other bottles. The 'vacu' bit comes from the fact that the blood bottles are filled with a vacuum which is released as blood starts to fill the bottles. The collection device attaches either to a winged collection needle (or 'butterfly') or directly to a needle (which may or may not have a flashback indicator).

This is currently considered the best method for blood collection as it protects the user from exposure to body fluids and also there is less risk of sending a haemolysed sample as the blood immediately hits the preservatives in the blood bottles.

Indications	Contraindications	Complications
• Too numerous to mention! See above	• No veins available – proceed with caution in legs and feet • Mastectomy +/- axillary clearance – avoid this arm • Phlebitis – find another vein • Arteriovenous fistula (for dialysis) – avoid this arm • Concurrent intravenous ipsilateral infusion • End of life care pathway has been commenced	• Bleeding/ haematoma • Arterial puncture • Nerve injury (usually just manifests itself as a shriek from the patient which settles when the needle's withdrawn) • Infection (rare)

Procedure

Make sure you have the **correct patient**, for the **correct procedure**. Check for any **allergies** (e.g. to the plaster you're going to put on at the end), and that you have confirmed the **indication;** excluded any **contraindications; explained** the procedure and taken **consent**. Now **wash your hands**!

Assemble all of your equipment on a sterile trolley away from the patient. You will need everything in the equipment textbox. Make sure that you **attach the plastic Vacutainer** collection port to the needle. Many trusts will have a phlebotomy trolley which you may be able to wheel to the bedside which is quite a handy surface to use. Others have plastic trays with a mini sharps bin which you can carry. Whatever you use – give it a clean with some disinfectant first.

Wash your hands and **put on your gloves**. **Position** your **patient**

Equipment you need (on a clean tray/trolley)

• Non-sterile gloves
• Tourniquet
• Vacutainer needle
• Vacutainer attachment
• Sterile gauze
• Tape
• Alcohol swab
• Sharps bin

comfortably. Some people find having the patient lying at 45° and resting their arm on a pillow makes it easier.

Apply your tourniquet about 4–5 cm above the point of venepuncture and ask the patient to **squeeze their fist** 10 times. **Gently rubbing** over the vein will help it to fill. Then with the index finger of your non dominant hand **palpate the vein** with your finger. The best vein will be a large vein that does not move when you palpate it and feels nice and compressible. Often an elderly patient will appear to have lovely veins over the back of their hand but you will notice that they are incredibly mobile, and most of their diameter is simply a thick wall with only a small lumen.

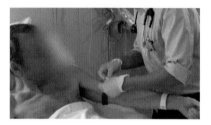

Securing the tourniquet 4–5 cm proximal to the venepuncture site

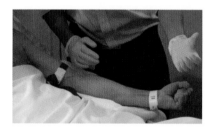

Asking the patient to make a fist

Once you have selected an adequate vein, **clean** it with an alcohol swab and **let it dry** for 30 seconds. Unsheathe your needle and with gentle pressure to stretch the adjacent skin with your non-dominant hand **advance the needle** into the vein. Just before you do so **warn the patient** of a 'sharp scratch'. With the vacutainer it's best to hold it between your thumb and index finger, and you can use your other fingers to stabilise

your hand. At the point where you think you are in the vein keep your hand as still as possible. Gently **insert the blood tubes** one-by-one into the collection set. Make sure to fill them in the correct draw order so that there is no cross-contamination of preservatives.

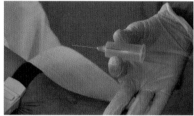

Holding the vacutainer attachment and needle correctly

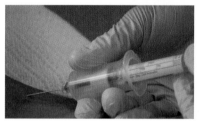

Inserting a blood bottle using the vacutainer system

Once you have finished taking blood **release the tourniquet. Remove the needle** and **apply pressure** with a gauze or cotton wool. Immediately **dispose of the sharp** – do not leave it in the tray, bed, floor or anywhere else. Remember, needle-sticks DO happen. You can then **tape the gauze down**. If you notice that pressure is not stopping the bleeding just check you haven't left the tourniquet on, it is an easy thing to forget.

Thank the patient and then most importantly **label** the blood bottles at the patient's bedside-do not wait to take them back to the nursing station, doctor's office or worse to another patient's bedside. Labelling errors can be disastrous, especially in the context of transfusion reactions.

Finally once the bottles have been labelled **fill out the request form** and send off the bloods to the laboratory. It's fairly obvious but make a note of which bloods you have taken as you will need to check them later.

Other methods

As mentioned earlier many people use a simple needle and syringe. In this case the method is exactly the same aside from the actual part where you take the blood. Once you have entered the vein you simply draw back the syringe to collect as much blood as required. The main benefit of this technique is that you can quickly reposition the needle and you can take as much blood as you need. Once you have taken blood you then need to get it into the tubes. You can either pierce the rubber tops with the needle or can flip off the tops of the blood bottles and squirt the blood in. The risk of the former method is a needle stick risk and of the latter method is that there can be contamination (for example of EDTA) into other tubes and the labs will reject the blood sample. You must also make sure that you have

properly fixed the top of the blood tubes back otherwise you will make a mess … Again we should reiterate that this method is discouraged.

The butterfly is many people's favourite. The butterfly is manoeuvrable, you can easily reposition and you instantly see a flashback. In addition you are handling the blood tubes well away from the needle which makes it much less fiddly, for instance if you're using a Vacutainer, exchanging the different blood bottles can be done without also inadvertently jiggling the needle. The butterfly can be attached to either a Vacutainer or a syringe.

Blood bottles

It's worth briefly mentioning blood bottles. There's no 'universal' colour coding for blood bottles but most trusts that use the Vacutainer method will use the same coloured bottles. The 'main' colours that you will use daily are (in the correct draw order):

Light blue which contains citrate for all your clotting tests. It is important to note that this tube **must** be filled exactly to the line otherwise it will be discarded.

Gold containing a serum separator gel for the main biochemistry tests.

Lavender containing EDTA for full blood count

Pink EDTA sample for group and save and subsequent crossmatch.

Grey. This fluoride tube is used for measuring serum glucose.

One further tip to note is that you should check with your trust their labelling protocols. Some trusts use electronic labelling where you can print a barcode whereas others require you to laboriously hand write all the bottles. Many trusts will have different labelling rules for a group and save sample and most will insist they are handwritten whether labels are available or not. Filling blood cultures bottles is slightly different (see above, Chapter 8: Blood Cultures).

Request forms

As you know the request form instructs the laboratory which tests need to be carried out. Some trusts employ electronic request forms whereas others still use old-fashioned paper. Whatever method is used it's crucial that it's completed correctly with the correct patient details including name, date of birth and hospital number as a minimum.

In addition to this the clinical indication needs to be documented. This is impor-

tant for a number of reasons. Firstly the lab needs to know the clinical context of the result – for example is an INR of 3 a normal result for a patient on warfarin or are they dangerously auto-anticoagulated from liver failure? Secondly many labs have strict criteria for which tests can be carried out in which circumstances – with careful correct documentation your test is more likely to get done. You should be able to justify what clinical reason there is for this test. If you cannot think of one then it should not have been requested. Worse you may find a result that you might have to act on or don't understand. And of course it's a waste of money and is painful for the patient to be bled when it's not indicated.

Check the request form in your trust and that you understand it. If you forget to request a test but remember later then don't worry, with most labs you can call them up within a few hours and they can simply add the test on.

OSCE checklist

- Assembles equipment correctly
- Applies tourniquet
- Positions arm correctly
- Cleans venepuncture site
- Holds needle correctly
- Warns about a 'sharp scratch'
- Inserts needle at appropriate angle
- Inserts blood bottle
- Successfully collects blood
- Releases tourniquet
- Withdraws needle and applies pressure
- Safely disposes of sharp
- Appropriately places dressing
- Labels samples correctly
- Completes request form
- Washes hands
- Thanks patient

43 Venesection

Video Time | 2 mins 54 s

Overview

Venesection is simply the removal of blood from a patient. This chapter will focus on the removal of blood for treatment purposes.

Therapeutic blood-letting has been in practice for thousands of years. Removal of blood was used originally to balance the bodily humours (other practices included inducing vomiting or promoting diuresis). Although the concepts of humours are no longer in favour, venesection is still an important treatment for a number of conditions.

Essentially any condition with a **raised level of haemoglobin** (polycythaemia) can be treated with venesection. This could be due to a primary polycythaemia (polycythaemia rubra vera) or secondary polycythaemia. Other conditions where venesection is indicated include those causing iron overload, such as hereditary haemochromatosis and those requiring exchange transfusion.

The process of venesection itself is a simple procedure; however, it is one that is not that often performed by junior doctors. The bulk of the work is performed by haematology trainees or specialist haematology nurses. Despite this there will be occasions when the junior doctor will be expected to venesect, so it's worth knowing.

As a rule of thumb, venesection of 1 unit should lower a patient's haemoglobin by 1 unit but it's always best to confirm this with a **formal laboratory haemoglobin**. The amount to venesect should be guided by the haematologist. In addition some patients require normovolaemic venesection in which case a bag of saline can be run in whilst you venesect – again check first with the experts.

How to Perform Clinical Procedures, First Edition. Matthew Stephenson, Joshua Shur and John Black.
© 2013 John Wiley & Sons, Ltd. Published 2013 by John Wiley & Sons, Ltd.

Procedure

Make sure you have the **correct patient**, for the **correct procedure**. Check for any **allergies**, and that you have confirmed the **indication;** excluded any **contra-indications; explained** the procedure and taken **consent**. Now **wash your hands**!

Assemble all of your equipment on a sterile trolley away from the patient. You will need everything in the equipment textbox.

Equipment you need (on a sterile tray/trolley)

- Blood collection set
- Tourniquet or sphygmomanometer and blood pressure cuff
- Inco
- Surgical tape
- Sterile pack
- Gauze
- Chlorhexidine containing alcohol swabs
- Sterile gloves
- Local anaesthetic such as 1% lidocaine (if the patient requires it)
- Clean metal trolley for your equipment

The only procedure specific piece of equipment is the blood collection set – if you're in doubt where to find one give the haematology department a call! Many patients who are venesected undergo the procedure regularly and may be more familiar than you with it, but as always it's good practice to explain the procedure. Some patients may know which vein is best to use, or which they prefer – always ask them first.

Get the patient **comfortable** for the procedure, preferably reclining in a chair –

fainting during this procedure is not unheard of! You can prop up their arm on a cushion and place an 'inco' pad underneath, this will make it more comfy for them and easier for you to perform the procedure.

A **simple tourniquet** can be placed, or sometimes more comfortable for the patient is to use a **blood pressure cuff** and 'sphyg'. Inflating to 40 to 60 mmHg will be more than enough; you only want to occlude the veins. The pressure is maintained until the desired volume of blood is collected.

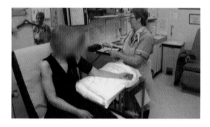

The patient resting comfortably with a sphygmomanometer to just above venous pressure

The procedure is carried out using an **aseptic technique** and ideally sterile gloves should be worn. The skin overlying the vein is sterilised with a chlorhexidine containing alcohol swab for 30 seconds. Leave the site to dry for approximately 30–60 seconds. Do not wipe the area dry.

As the blood collection pack needle has been described as a 'drain pipe' some people like to use **local anaesthetic**. As you all know, intravenous administration of local anaesthetic is *not* recommended and so if you do want to use some local, be very careful to raise a bleb just next to the vein, rather than in its lumen.

Once the patient is ready you need to 'unfurl' the venesection pack. As we mentioned earlier it comes with a needle attached and it will also have an extra piece of 'side' tubing that will allow you to take blood samples.

Insert the venesection needle into the vein, preferably the antecubital or a forearm vein. Once it starts to fill with blood try not to move it around as it can be uncomfortable. Some people find gently taping the needle in place to the arm stops it moving around and disrupting the blood flow. Positioning the collection pack below the patient's level facilitates blood flow into the bag. Also very gentle adjustment of the needle angle can help get the blood moving if it's quite sluggish.

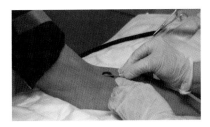

The venesection needle is large bore, don't be surprised if a drop of blood leaks out around the side

If you wish to collect samples whilst venesecting, clamp off the main line (in the video this clamp is white) and open the tube to the collection set (in the video this clamp is blue). Snap the tubing

just proximal to the collection set and it should fill with blood. Once you have discarded two bottles you may collect samples as required. To restart the venesection simply close the clamp to the collection set and open the main line again.

After 5–10 minutes the venesection should be complete. In practise there is no *exact* amount of blood to be venesected, but the bag should not be completely full with blood – with practise you can get an accurate judge of how much to take off.

Prior to removing the needle, deflate the cuff and clamp the line. Once the needle is removed, gently place a dressing over the venepuncture site. It will need a decent amount of pressure due to the size of the puncture site. Inspect the site for haemostasis before applying a firm bandage. The blood collected from therapeutic venesection should be disposed of for incineration. Like giving blood – don't suggest your patient plays a game of rugby after the procedure. Patients should be advised not to drive either. A good 5–10 minutes rest and then gentle mobilisation is advisable. Finally, document the procedure in the notes.

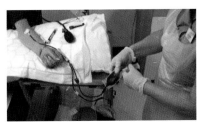

The side arm of this collection pack has a port to which you can attach a Vacutainer to take off your blood samples

Appendix I: Consent

'It is well established that, as a general rule, the performance of a medical operation upon a person without his or her consent is unlawful, as constituting both the crime of battery and the tort of trespass to the person.'

Lord Goff 1990

Introduction

Consenting the patient means that irritating step of getting them to sign that big yellow form before you're let loose on them, doesn't it? Well unfortunately that's how it's often interpreted, and practised. Consent to many may sound like a boring dry subject, but if you're going to be a doctor, you'd better get interested in it, and fully understand it. If you don't, a career's worth of disgruntled patients, lawsuits, and even (theoretically) a spell in one of Her Majesty's buildings, awaits you. And I don't mean one of the palaces. This by no means will be a comprehensive review of consent – it would take up several tomes – this is a brief whistle stop tour.

First, issues of consent for procedures fall into two broad categories: those patients who **can consent for themselves**, and **those who can't**. Furthermore consent can be divided up into: **implied consent** and **expressed consent**.

Implied consent means that by virtue of a patient's actions, you can fairly confidently say that they would agree to what you're about to do. For instance, if a patient turns up to the hospital to have his blood taken, you can quite confidently imply that he is giving consent to it. He doesn't need to sign a big yellow form. Ditto with many of the procedures in this book. Nevertheless, it's right even with the most basic procedure to simply ask the patient if it's ok to proceed.

How to Perform Clinical Procedures, First Edition. Matthew Stephenson, Joshua Shur and John Black.
© 2013 John Wiley & Sons, Ltd. Published 2013 by John Wiley & Sons, Ltd.

Expressed consent therefore is a clear and unmistakeable statement that the patient agrees to have something done. It can be either **verbal** or **written**. In the majority of procedures verbal consent is all that is required. You don't for instance expect a patient to sign a form if you're going to put a cannula in their arm. A court of law would not expect that. It's the more invasive procedures, the ones that might come as a bit more of a surprise to the patient and particularly those with a risk profile, that require written, signed consent. It's largely up to your common sense to distinguish which are which, but this is also dictated by individual trust policies. For instance, some trusts will expect a signed consent form to be completed for a central line insertion, other will accept verbal consent. The way things are going, more and more procedures require signed consent forms. If in doubt, fill one out.

Issues of consent affect surgeons significantly and it's within surgery that most of the case law has evolved but the principles are the same.

Assessment of capacity

To decide which group your patient falls into, you need to decide if they have capacity to make decisions about their treatment. The first principle is that you **assume all patients over the age of 16 to have the required capacity** unless shown otherwise.

According to the **Mental Capacity Act (MCA) 2005**, a patient will not have capacity if he is unable to do one or more of the following:

1 **Understand** the information relevant to the decision
2 **Retain** that information
3 **Weigh up** the **pros and cons** related to the decision
4 **Communicate** the decision

Often, the above is not completely clear cut and everyone, including the courts, accept this. What is important is that you make reasonable decisions and

document clearly in the notes anything that may seem contentious and how you've come to your conclusion. Furthermore, a patient may have the capacity to make decisions about one thing, but not another, or this may vary over time.

Patients with capacity

Assessment of capacity is just the first step for this group, there are two other vital ingredients to obtaining consent. The three components are:

1 The patient has **capacity** (see above)
2 The patient is **fully informed** about the procedure
3 The consent is **voluntary**

In other words, it's no good getting a perfectly competent intelligent patient to consent to a procedure unless you have fully informed them of the nature of the procedure, the pros and cons and the alternatives. Equally, consent isn't valid if you've twisted their arm because you really wanted to do their procedure, or you misrepresent the value of an alternative option or the patient is being bullied into it by a caring relative.

This second point is a bit sticky – just how much do you tell the patient about the risks of a procedure? For this we must look to some **English case law**. You may have heard of the **Bolam (and Bolitho) tests**. As Mr Justice McNair put it in Bolam in 1957:

I myself would prefer to put it this way, that he is not guilty of negligence if he has acted in accordance with a practice accepted as proper by a responsible body of medical men skilled in that particular art. I do not think there is much difference in sense. It is just a different way of expressing the same thought. Putting it the other way round, a man is not negligent, if he is acting in accordance with such a practice, merely because there is a body of opinion who would take a contrary view. At the same time, that does not mean that a medical man can obstinately and pig-headedly carry on with some old technique if it has been proved to be contrary to what is really substantially the whole of informed medical opinion. Otherwise you might get men today saying: 'I do not believe in anaesthetics. I do not believe in antiseptics. I am going to continue to do my surgery in the way it was done in the eighteenth century.' That clearly would be wrong.

This applied to consent in that a doctor would be expected to tell his patient about whatever risks a responsible body of doctors would tell their patients in the same circumstances.

In other words, if Doctor X never warned his hernia repair patients about the risk of chronic groin pain and a patient sues Doctor X because he didn't warn him, Dr X could get away with it if he could find a group of his mates who wouldn't have warned the patient in those circumstances either, *providing* that those mates held a view that was capable of withstanding logical analysis; a decision which would ultimately fall to be made by the Court.

This dominated the legal scene for a long time – and amounted to telling the patient about all of the common potential risks – but the crucial question has been: how common does a risk have to be to tell the patient? In the case of **Sidaway v Bethlem Royal Hospital** (1985), the claimant failed in her lawsuit against her neurosurgeon for not telling her about the 1% risk of paraplegia (which she unfortunately developed) during a cervical cord decompression. The court felt that the surgeon was not under a duty to warn the patient about remote side effects, they felt a risk of 10% was a reasonable cut off. In the case of **Pearce v United Bristol** (1999), the pregnant defendant was overdue by about two weeks and requested an induction or caesarean section. She was advised by her consultant to proceed with a natural delivery but this resulted in a stillbirth. She lost her case because the risk of proceeding with a natural birth was only in the order of 0.1–0.2% but the court did contend that doctors should **err on the side of generosity** in giving information to their patients.

Importantly in the Pearce case, the Court found that if there was a significant risk which would affect the judgement of **a reasonable patient**, then in the normal course it is the responsibility of a doctor to inform the patient of that significant risk so that the patient can determine for him or herself as to what course s/he should adopt. However this should only be done if the doctor believes that the disclosure of such information would not cause the patient significant harm or distress – the 'therapeutic privilege'.

The next big case to challenge the received wisdom of risk was **Chester v Afshar** (2004). Mrs Chester suffered neurological injury following neurosurgical intervention for her lower back and claimed to have never been warned about it, the risk being in the order of 1–2%. She won. A precedent had been set in which serious complications, even if they were unlikely, should be raised with the patient.

As if that didn't make it complicated enough, there was then the case of **Birch v UCL Hospital** (2008). Mrs Birch was admitted with a third nerve palsy and underwent a diagnostic angiogram to look for a cerebral aneurysm. She was appropriately counselled about the risks of the angiogram. She suffered a stroke, sued the hospital, and won – why? Because she wasn't told about the

alternatives, and the pros and cons of the alternatives (and in particular an MRI which would not have had the risk of a stroke) so she was found to have been denied an opportunity to properly weigh the comparative risks and benefits of competing procedures.

So there has been a paradigm shift away from warning patients about risks that seem **reasonable to the doctor** (or body of doctors), to warning the patient about risks that would seem **reasonable to the patient**. In other words, a 0.5% risk of causing ischaemic orchitis following a primary inguinal hernia repair may not seem too troubling to you as the surgeon, but if you were the patient, you may have wanted to know. What's more – have you told your patient that whilst you can offer an open inguinal hernia repair, Mr X down the road could do it laparoscopically (and all that that might entail)?

In short – consent, even for a patient with capacity, can be very, very thorny. But in general you are far safer by telling the patient more, rather than less, even if the risk is small. And by the way, what if you don't actually write down on the consent form or in the notes that you've warned the patient that the varicose veins might come back? Who do you think the civil courts are going to believe – you or the patient? Sorry, but it will be the patient almost all of the time. Remember civil courts need only prove, on the 'balance of probabilities' (not 'beyond all reasonable doubt' as in criminal courts) and who will the court consider is more likely to remember what you said on that day three years ago when you saw the patient in day surgery? The patient who's only had one operation in her life and for whom it was a major event, or you, who's done hundreds of operations since then and can't even remember her name?

So essentially, it's not about getting that patient to scribble a mark on a yellow form – it's a matter of confirming they have capacity to make that decision, ensuring they are fully informed of the procedure and all it entails including the alternatives and finally letting them think and cogitate on it. The scribbling on the 'form' is merely evidence that you said what you did, when you did – it is not 'consent'.

Patients without capacity

But what about patients who you think don't have capacity to make decisions? The **Mental Capacity Act (MCA) 2005**, which came into force in October 2007 pulled together much of the ad-hoc case law that had accumulated over the years. It was designed to codify the underlying principles to protect patients who lack capacity. Let's use an example from surgery, the principles are the same. Say, for instance, a man with Down's syndrome with associated severe learning disabilities comes to see you in clinic – he has an inguinal hernia (this isn't an emergency). The patient has no living relatives and no other legally recognised directive. In the past,

if the doctor felt it was in the best interests of the patient to have his hernia repaired, he would proceed.

So what should you do now? Firstly, is it possible that the patient **may regain his capacity** and you must consider if the decision for treatment is **delayable** until then? If so you should wait, but this usually isn't the case. Secondly, you must **enable the patient** as much as possible in taking part in the decision making process – even if you can't get a full and clear idea of what they would want, the little information you can still glean is useful. Thirdly, you must consider any **premorbid wishes expressed** – either verbally or written in for instance an **advance directive** (a legally recognised statement made by the patient when he/she has capacity, to be invoked if he/she loses capacity) or if the patient has appointed a **lasting power of attorney** (someone who the patient appointed when they had capacity, to take on such decisions in the event that they lose capacity, it replaced the **enduring power of attorney**). Fourthly, you must take the views of those closest to the **patient** (even if not appointed as lasting powers of attorney) – usually the family, but also healthcare professionals. Normally this is sufficient to form a decision, but that decision to treat must be a reasonable one and made only after, and on the basis of, this holistic assessment of the patient's interests. It must be written in the notes in full with a thorough explanation of why and how the decision was reached. There is usually a special form in your hospital to fill in too. This should be enough to make a safe, considered decision in the best interests of the patient and keep you out of trouble.

But what happens if the patient has no family? They live in a nursing home and all their friends and family are dead. They have no advance directive and there's no lasting power of attorney. They are unbefriended. Meet the **Independent Mental Capacity Advocate (IMCA)**. These are non-medical individuals who you must get in contact with in these circumstances; your hospital will have a local IMCA service. They will arrange to meet with you to discuss the best interests of the patient, the IMCA representing what one would hope to be the best interests of the patient. In other words, the paternalism of days gone has vanished – doctor does not necessarily know best. Ignoring this would be extremely unwise.

Special circumstances
Emergencies
In the emergency situation where the patient has capacity to make decisions, you can obviously proceed as you normally would, although the steps are bound to be quicker and you, the patient and the court would accept that their time for cogitation would be limited. Worrying about being sued over this must not delay a vital procedure. In emergencies, what needs to be done, gets done. The gloves come off (or on, to be more precise). For the patient without capacity to make decisions, which may be an unconscious patient or one with long-term lack of capacity, you must act in the patient's best interests and provide only that treatment which is necessary (until capacity can be re-established) – in true traditional paternalist style – and without further ado. In fact, many of the procedures in this book will fall into this context.

Paediatrics
In the 16–17 year old category, patients can consent for procedures, but strictly they can't refuse them against medical advice if this would not be in their best interests. Such rare situations require great tact and care. In the rarest of situations, an application to court may be necessary. In the under-16 category, in general, patients are deemed to be children and their parents must consent for them and act in the child's best interests. However, the case of *Gillick v West Norfolk* (1985) in which a child was prescribed contraception without the knowledge of her mother set a precedent. If the minor is able to understand the information, in much the same way as an adult – they are deemed '**Gillick competent**' – that is, they are treated as an adult and can consent as such. The decision is reached on a case by case basis and will require you to consider the mental, emotional and chronological age of the child, their ability to understand and their ability to appreciate the consequences of their decision.

Summary

- **All patients over the age of 16 have the capacity** to make decisions unless shown otherwise
- A patient must be able to **understand**, **retain** and **weigh up** the information and be able to **communicate** it
- In a patient with capacity, consent must be **fully informed** and **voluntary** to be legally recognised
- Inform patients of all the **common risks** and any **potentially serious risks**, even if the chances are small. Err on the side of more, rather than less
- The **Mental Capacity Act 2005** changed the management of patients without capacity
- **Advance Directives** and **Lasting Power of Attorney** need to be considered in decision making in those without capacity
- If in doubt, appoint an **Independent Mental Capacity Advocate** (IMCA)
- In **emergencies**, if in doubt, act in what you see as the **best interests** of the patient
- Patients aged **16-17 can consent** to treatment but **can't refuse** it
- Patients **under 16 can consent** to treatment if they are **Gillick competent.**

Appendix II: How To Be a Great F1

Rosemary Chester

This chapter focuses on how to be a good FY1 or House Officer in old money. This can be one of the most *life-affirming* years of your life. However, passing through it is by no means your golden ticket, and as with most milestone things in life, you just have to *do it*. Hopefully, however, there are some useful pointers and tips on how to ease through this tempestuous transitional period of your life.

Aside from the realisation of having actual money to spend (after rather begrudgingly surrendering student loan repayments, income tax, pension contributions, mess fees and hospital car park fees), working at the front-line of the hospital is usually exciting, eye-opening, inspiring, challenging, at times harrowing, but definitely one of the most positive times of your life.

So welcome to the family! Here are a few tips to help you along the way. Every individual will have a completely different experience, but hopefully you'll find the advice here useful as you take your first tentative steps into the world of being a *real* doctor, with a lifetime of responsibility and clenched buttocks.

Before you start…

At some point before you've possibly even taken your finals, you will receive a package from your prospective employer full of scary documents called 'contracts' and 'pension plans' etc. I would recommend reading through this paperwork thoroughly, getting all the necessary documents together and making copies of things like passports, driving licenses, GMC certificates, and degree certification. You will need them at every hospital you work in so it's best to have them saved to your computer to avoid the kafuffle of scanning them each time. It's at this point also that you should start to

How to Perform Clinical Procedures, First Edition. Matthew Stephenson, Joshua Shur and John Black.
© 2013 John Wiley & Sons, Ltd. Published 2013 by John Wiley & Sons, Ltd.

accumulate all of your certificates and paperwork into one folder, your **portfolio**, which will evolve as you progress through your training.

The BMA offer a **contract service** where they will read through the contract and make sure it's appropriate. The BMA are worth joining early on if you're not already a member. The vast majority of new doctors have no major problems with the trust employing them, but if you do have a problem, the BMA are actually pretty powerful and resourceful when it come to solving employment issues. If you're not a member of a **trade union**, you're on your own if you do run into trouble. The NHS is likely to undergo major structural change over the next few years and this will almost certainly include contractual alterations for junior doctors for an increasingly outdated contract. Make sure you have someone fighting your corner. Most problems though can be resolved locally with your employer. The Medical Staffing Department, for example, expect questions, and most offer a prompt, and *occasionally* helpful response!

Some NHS Trusts require you to complete a series of online e-learning modules prior to starting work such as blood transfusion competencies, child protection, equality and diversity etc. Save copies of the certificates as you may need this evidence at induction.

After the haze and hangover of graduation ceremonies and parties are over, you should be asked to complete a period of **induction and F1 shadowing**. You may also be asked to do some mandatory **courses** such as Immediate Life Support (ILS), Acute Life-Threatening Events: Recognition and Treatment (ALERT) and other simulation training. Do try to complete these as early as possible as they can be a real headache to get done at the end of the year before portfolio sign-off, and unfortunately you do need to have completed them in order to avoid repeating the year. Really you should have done them as early in the year as possible, as they should be helpful for your clinical work.

Induction is a series of *exciting* lectures about fire safety, record-keeping, governance *blah blah blah* but in amongst the dross, there are usually some useful hints and tips, especially on things like death certification and 'how to look up bloods or perform electronic discharges' which you should *definitely* stay awake for … this will be your LIFE for the next year! Induction also gives you the opportunity to meet your fellow F1s, and usually a chance to network with other junior colleagues already in post who can offer all sorts of advice on the jobs you'll be stepping into and the consultants you'll be stepping up to.

Whilst **shadowing**, it's easy to forget to find out all of the mundane but essential things and get lost in seeing the patients you will be taking over the care of. But my advice would be to find out how to use the blood collection systems, where to go to request urgent scans, how to order other investigations like ECGs, ECHOs, and endoscopies. If you can, introduce yourself to your consultant/clinical supervisor and find out what they expect from you, their own rota, their phone extension and possibly mobile number, and especially where and when to meet them on that first Wednesday of August, '*Black Wednesday*'! Introduce yourself to the senior sister/s on the wards you will be working on, and as many nurses as possible. You may not remember all their names now, but believe me, make a good impression and they will literally be *life-savers* when you need it the most. They go through this process every August and know the workings of the hospital better than anyone. They know you will be nervous and they want to help you as much as possible to keep their ward working smoothly, and most importantly of all, safely. So try, at all costs to keep them on side. They are usually easily bought with a bag of wine gums, or Haribo tangtastic mix.

First day nerves

Turn up early on your first day. If you live on-site don't leave it until the last minute to crawl out of bed! Typically, with anything like this, it's the people that live the closest that get in the latest. If you're driving, be aware of how busy it can be around the hospital first thing in the morning – finding a space in the staff car park can be a nightmare, so leave plenty of time!

Dress like you're going to visit your elderly, easily offended, judgmental grandma. For the male contingent, this is relatively simple. A smart shirt and trousers will suffice, with a pair of smart shoes. Ties are banned in many trusts now, due to their alleged infection control risk, despite the absolute absence of meaningful evidence. Your consultant (if of the 'old boy' descent) may continue to defy these laws, and insist on waging war with the infection control brigade, which at times can be entertaining to watch, but as a junior just starting, you're powerless. If ties are allowed, be sure to tuck it into your shirt or wear a tie clip, because it's irritating when it dangles into an open wound. Many patients, especially older ones, really appreciate their doctors looking smart, that is, wearing a tie, so if you're allowed to, there's no reason why not. For females, it's a little trickier. Basically you still want to make a good impression, but nothing too controversial. Try to avoid plunging neck lines, and make sure the hair is under control. White coats have also been banished NHS-wide from clinical areas for similar spurious infection control reasons.

There may be a queue at switchboard to **collect your bleep**. Find out beforehand which number you're looking for and it will make the process much quicker for everyone. Sometimes, however, you have to get your bleep from the outgoing F1 who of course has left the trust by now and entrusted the bleep to a colleague who left it with a friend, who left it with another friend who thinks they last saw it on a pile of old copies of *TV Guide* in the doctor's mess.

On your **first clinical day**, go to your ward, print off the updated list for the day, and then find out from the nurses if there have been any issues overnight with the patients, and if there are any potential discharges looming. Read through the notes of your patients, and familiarise yourself with any new patients on the ward that may come under your care, then you can dazzle your consultant on Day 1 with your knowledge of their case when he/she arrives. You've got to play the game.

You should have found out from your outgoing F1 how your consultant likes to conduct the **ward round**, that is, with the notes trolley, whether he/she wants his/her own list etc. Get everything ready for their arrival, and keep a bunch of blood forms and x-ray requests handy to complete as you go round. Every consultant usually has a few pet topics they like to discuss with new doctors, or pet investigations they like ordered for each patient. Try to learn these idiosyncracies before starting.

DO NOT LOSE YOUR LIST! Not only is it a confidentiality issue if left lying around in the canteen, but also your list is your *lifeline*, especially in the first few weeks. Losing lists which are then found by Mrs Bloggs on the Number 57 bus, has resulted in serious disciplinary action for doctors before. Make your own code for how to denote whether jobs have been done, tests requested etc. (I like to put a square next to a job, if I have requested the investigation, then I put a diagonal line though it, if the test has been completed but the results aren't back then I shade half of it in, and if the job/results are completed then I shade the whole thing in – just an idea, but it worked for me.)

Make a note of any extension numbers you will need frequently, for example microbiology, haematology, biochemistry, radiology, medical/surgical reg bleeps etc. A '**useful number' list** is invaluable and may already be on your patient list courtesy of your predecessor and may just need some updating. Crucially, make sure you have the numbers of the people you may need help from urgently.

In most places, your F2s/SHOs will be completing their own induction on 'Black Wednesday' so you may be the only junior on your team. Your firms and the ward staff know this; many more senior people take annual leave just to avoid it! But jobs still need to be completed regardless of it being your first day amidst a depleted workforce. Start early. Be prepared, hangover-free and fully caffeinated if necessary. Do your best – **ask the nurses for help** where possible, and if you have any concerns regarding patients then contact your registrar or consultant early rather than sitting on the problem… it will only get bigger!

If you're unlucky enough to have a patient 'go off' badly on your first day, then get the Outreach Service on board early (most hospitals have these now), and ask the nursing staff to contact your senior immediately, regardless of whether they are in clinic. Start with the basics… ABCDE, take bloods, get IV access and start fluids, get portable X-rays and blood gases as appropriate, and if your senior can't attend, page the on-call one.

If you're **on-call** on your first day or night (as I was) then it can be *incredibly* daunting. I contacted the other F1 on-call and we decided to stay in close contact, and share any jobs that came up, and if possible to attend sick patients together. You certainly can't complete all on-calls this way, but on our first day having someone else there gave us a bit more confidence. Make use of your peers despite their mirrored relative inexperience.

You will learn to prioritise quickly on the on-calls, especially if they are ward-based. Nurses will call you for fluids / venflons / sick patients / warfarin dosing. Obviously all of these are important, but do ask questions – if it's 9 pm and the patient needs a venflon for their 8 am antibiotics then it's not your priority. You will most probably have more pressing issues. Many nurses can cannulate, so if you're snowed under, consider asking them (politely) to find a nurse to try. If you have the time however, you should do as many of these procedures as possible yourself – that's what the rest of this book is all about. If your on-call is within the admissions department, then this is the perfect arena to learn how to manage acute patients, do lots of procedures and also to get a lot of your assessments done. So roll up your sleeves, and get in the mix!

The hospital at night can be a scary place. All too often you face the harrowing task of a skeleton team looking after the entire joint, and an on-call that can be as busy as the day take. Don't panic, *prioritise* your tasks. There is usually a team of site nurse practitioners on to offer some support, so don't be afraid to use them. Remember, you still have a medical and surgical registrar usually on-site, and a couple of 'SHOs' who have been through the experience. Make use of them if necessary.

Regarding **calls from nurses**, these shape much of the way your day will play out. The more organised you are, the less often nurses will have to call you to write that discharge summary or rewrite the drug chart. But however organised you are, much of your job will still consist of responding to nurse requests. One of the big secrets to having a successful F1 (and future career) is quite simple – be nice to nurses! The F1 that graduates and adopts a cocky know-it-all attitude is not only deluded but will have no end of struggles with the nurses. Nurses are often an invaluable source of help and support to you, aside from their main role as being nurses.

You will no doubt overhear colleagues moaning about such and such nurse for always paging about seemingly trivial matters. Without trying to sound too high and mighty, I suggest you try and see things slightly differently. You both have different skill sets. Nurses wouldn't mock you for asking them to dress a wound because you weren't sure how to, for instance.

Handover

Make sure you know where to receive handover, and listen carefully. Take heed of any sick patients you have been given a heads up about, and make sure to write down their details and location. Handover should be a strictly bleep free half an hour to an hour meeting (obviously dependent on the number of patients) in many trusts. The hospital staff are aware of this and should not be bleeping you during this period. Handover is paramount to patient safety. Finally, prepare yourself for a night of continual bleeping! Answer every bleep and triage the urgency, writing down the details of the call. If you do miss a bleep, don't be alarmed, as the person will undoubtedly bleep again if the matter is pressing. For example, you may be tied up with a sick patient.

Many people bang on about handover and sometimes it might seem like overkill, but in reality handing over information is crucial to the smooth running of the hospital. The reason is simple: handover is *so* much more important than it ever used to be as it occurs *so* much more frequently that it used to.

Since those politicians in Brussels decided that we can't work 'proper' weeks, shifts have been chopped, staggered, overlapped, and *banded* all so we don't tire ourselves out. The result is a variety of handovers throughout the day, some informal, some formal. Gone are the days of 24-hour on-calls when the house officer would see through their patient's first day in hospital, and then become part of the team that looks after them under their supervising consultant. Now typically on-call shifts will occur twice-a-day with handovers in between. What this means for you is that you will have to receive information, and relay it over. If you are covering 'wards' then there will undoubtedly be a flurry of calls around 5-o-clock as the day team leave for the pub/golf/wherever. Handover can also occur before the weekend, whereby the weekend team will have to follow up any urgent jobs that have been left for them.

In general when handing over information: be clear, be specific (not just 'please review this patient'), and have clear instructions for what to do with abnormal results. Include a brief history and ceiling for escalation.

Things to hand over
- **Important blood results** that may need chasing with a **clear** plan of action with how to respond to them, that is, Mr Smith on Milton ward has been bleeding. If their Hb on Saturday comes back as <8 please can you prescribe 2 units of blood. They have been crossmatched and the blood is ready just in case.

- **Sick patients** that may need review. such as, Mrs Jones has been quite unwell today with sepsis. Please can you review her this evening and if her urine output is still poor increase her fluid rate. If she still doesn't respond then she may need higher level care. The HDU team are aware of the patient and I have discussed this with the medical registrar.
- **Patients that can go home** (this will be directed by your Reg/Consultant), that is, Mr Bloggs can go home tomorrow if his CRP<50 and he is walking. His electronic discharge has been completed and his meds are ready for collection. I have requested the phlebotomists to bleed him in the morning so please just check these have come back.
- **Important scan results** that are yet to come back, that is, Mrs Wilson had a fall earlier and is a bit tender over her ribs. Her saturations have been a little bit low since so we have requested a CXR. Please can you check for any signs of pneumothorax and if there is one escalate as appropriate.

Things not to hand over
- I haven't finished my ward round and it's 5-o-clock. Please can you see these patients… (this is not a job for the on-call!)
- Can you check these bloods for these patients… (if there are no reasons as to why they need to be done out of hours. Only bloods with real clinical need should be checked out of hours)

- Pretty much any job where you haven't done the basics/don't know your patients.

In addition the following jobs should NEVER be left for the weekend/on-call team. (If you're caught doing this expect the wrath of your colleagues!)
- Warfarin dosing (unless the patient is being re-warfarinised and the dose may need to be altered depending on an INR result).
- Drug charts that may need re-writing. These should have been anticipated and done in advance.
- Discharge summaries (should have been anticipated).

To ensure proper handover many trusts have developed handover proformas to ensure it's done properly – if they exist use them.

When you have made a mistake

We have put this section of the appendix in not to scare you but just to offer some advice from the author's own experiences. As humans we **make mistakes**, and unfortunately not infrequently.

If you make a mistake the first thing to do is to take a deep breath. Check that the patient is OK and that clinical care has not been affected – often it will not have been. Document what has happened in the notes and inform your seniors. Sometimes an incident form should be completed. Don't worry, it's not a blame exercise it's simply so that we can learn from our experiences. If clinical care has been affected then your immediate priority must be to make sure that they get the correct management. Inform your seniors and proceed as above.

Don't take it personally, use it as an opportunity to reflect: believe it or not reflection can improve practice. Think about what happened, how it affected the patient, how it affected yourself and how your practice will change. Remember it can be an extra sheet for your portfolio! Don't let it knock your confidence, but use it as an opportunity to be a better doctor.

Jumping through hoops

By which I mean of course, the dreaded e-Portfolio. Learn to love it. So… a quick breakdown (subject to change by the UKFPO):

Within each 4 month rotation you must complete:

1 x initial meeting with educational/ clinical supervisor

At least *2 x mini-CEX* (short case – usually with a consultant, registrar, or CT/ST1 or above)

At least *2 x CBD* (long case – usually consultant/registrar only)

At least *1 x DOPS* (anyone competent in the procedure)

1 x *Clinical Supervisor report*

1 x end-of-placement meeting with educational supervisor

Within the year, you must also complete the following:

1 x Developing the Clinical Teacher – usually some sort of presentation to your peers with a consultant presence

demonstrating your ability to teach on a subject. If you have a weekly meeting within your firm then it would be a good idea to lead a teaching session within this and get it signed off.

1 x Multi-source feedback (360 assessment) – I would advise doing this in your very first placement, because if you don't get enough electronic forms back from the right ratio of people by the closing period then you will need to complete it again to pass…and it really isn't something you want to leave to the last minute because collecting people's email addresses actually takes quite a bit of time.

There are various other forms and questionnaires to fill out, as well as reflections and uploading certificates and evidence. It's worth spending a bit of time familiarising yourself with the ePortfolio early on, getting as many links to each aspect of the curriculum as possible, and understanding the layout – because your consultant almost certainly won't know how to fill out forms and sometimes even how to log in, and you will need to *gently* guide them through this arduous task.

You also have a number of '*Core Procedures*' to complete. Don't fall into the trap of getting your friendly F2 to sign them all off for you – the person assessing you should be CT/ST1 or above and you should ideally get a variety of people to assess you. Again, get as many of these done early on, and plan which firms will be more amenable to certain procedures to avoid a last-minute panic to find a female patient to catheterise or someone to pass a nasogastric tube down.

Some consultants are easy to touch base with to get meetings and evidence signed off, but some are a nightmare to pin down. As with all things, the sooner you can meet with them, the less you have to worry about at the end of the year, so contact them/their secretary early to arrange a convenient space in their timetable. They understand you're busy, and if you can't make the appointment, simply ring and rearrange, but don't leave it until the last minute to make an appointment as you can guarantee that they will take three weeks' annual leave during the signoff deadline! If you have any problems, either with contacting your consultants or getting signoffs done in a timely fashion, contact your F1 lead.

On top of all of this, you need to obtain a minimum attendance of 70% at teaching, which can be extremely difficult if you are on busy banded placements all year. Liaise with your Postgraduate Centre to find out your percentage from March-time and see if you can attend F2 teaching to boost your attendance rating if necessary.

Summary

Remember you're not superhuman, although sometimes it feels like the world expects you to be. Help is out there if you need it, and you should never suffer in silence. Remember that you cannot do *everything*, it's sometimes not humanly possible to. If you haven't managed to write that referral yet that your boss asked you to, then just explain that you haven't had a chance and that you will do it as your next priority. Don't lie to your boss. Probity is taken seriously and if you're caught talking porkies then it will reflect very badly.

Remember 75% of being a good F1 is organisation and clerical work...if you can prioritise, delegate and get everything done efficiently then you will please your team and make yourself indispensible to them.

Get involved in the Doctor's Mess, get involved in your clinical work, and take opportunities to do audits/presentations/posters/publications. They will stand you in good stead for the rat race of getting the next training post. Believe it or not, hospital work will never be as new and exciting as it is the year you do your F1, so above all, enjoy it!

Appendix III: How To Be an Even Better F2

Stephanie Ball

First of all, let me briefly introduce myself. My name is Dr Stephanie Ball, and I'm currently bumbling my way through some dark hospital corridors in my new role as a Core Medical Trainee. I'm somewhere in the East Midlands deanery, not too far from Skegness apparently! Haven't made it to Butlin's yet, but just you wait till I get some annual leave…

Dr John Black is the other contributor to this chapter, and has recently embarked on Core Surgical Training in the London Deanery (South East Thames Rotation). We felt that united we broadly represent the training specialities (Medicine and Surgery). We shall aim to provide you with a good service, covering all bases on the F2 year and beyond, having recently both been through the application and interview process. To keep things simple, this chapter is written as first-person narrative despite a combined effort. It's just easier that way…

So … you are no longer a lowly F1. Congratulations on your promotion! A minor pay rise and lifetime of delegation awaits, and with it comes greater responsibility.

If you are anything like me, you will probably worry that you're as equally inept as you were this time last year, but don't worry – that just isn't true. You will be surprised at how much you have learnt via osmosis alone. All those ward rounds you've traipsed around on will have honed your management skills, and those nights spent waddling around the wards in your uncomfortable high heels will have made you an expert in that elusive skill coveted by medical students worldwide – cannulation. Things will come more naturally to you, and it should overall be a more enjoyable

How to Perform Clinical Procedures, First Edition. Matthew Stephenson, Joshua Shur and John Black.
© 2013 John Wiley & Sons, Ltd. Published 2013 by John Wiley & Sons, Ltd.

experience than when you first started out as an F1. However, as I've already mentioned – you now have extra duties and more is expected of you. You also have the looming threat of WHAT TO DO NEXT! … I'll come on to that part later.

Your role as an F2 doctor

I thought, in this section, it might be a good idea to summarise what is expected of you according to the UK Foundation Programme Office. I, in a rather obsessional manner, read the whole booklet. Crumbs! It's 86 pages long! That's a *lot* of recommendations. I won't include all of them here, and anyway, it's quite straightforward to see what you need to achieve by the end of the year if you look at the 'Foundation Curriculum' on your e-portfolio. You'll see there are a few extra bits you need to have done, in addition to what was required of you as an F1. Here are my Top 8 key points from reading through, along with my analysis of what the big dogs want:

1. Act with professionalism with patients and colleagues. Act as a role model, and where appropriate a leader for medical students and other junior doctors

Professionalism goes without saying. You should always act with integrity and transparency, and be appropriate with your peers, juniors, seniors and patients – hell, be nice to everyone! However, as an F2 you are now someone the juniors will want guidance from. As their most direct senior, you are ergo often the most approachable person for them when it comes to advice

(and failed cannulas, for that matter). Even if they aren't asking you questions, they will often observe how you write notes – or interact with a patient – in order to learn from you. Please remember what it was like when you were an F1, be kind and patient. New doctors are often petrified at the idea of cocking up, so give them a hand and help them find their feet. Try and remember that you were once thrust into this position. Saying this, if you yourself are uncertain about something, signpost them on to obtaining help from someone higher up the chain. A few times during my F2, I felt embarrassed about having to say 'I don't know' when an F1 or student asked me a question. But it's better to admit your uncertainties than try and blag something in order to save face, and ultimately make yourself look like an even bigger numpty than you actually are.

2. Delegates tasks, ensures they are completed, organises handover and task allocation within the team

This is one of the major transitions you make between F1 and F2 – you now get to **delegate**. This can make you feel quite uncomfortable to begin with – it feels strange not to be the ward *admin* and just do what you are told all day. You now need to engage your brain and make decisions. I didn't much like doling out tasks to begin with – I felt rather sheepish giving the F1s and medical students jobs to do and bossing them around. Some people are more natural leaders, or just lazy, than others, but task allocation and taking charge is an extremely important part of being a doctor. Imagine if a consultant went around taking his own bloods all day because he or she didn't want to trouble someone else! That would be ridiculous. It's your job to decide who does what, and to make sure things are divvied up fairly. It might be that after the ward round, you send the F1 to take some bloods whilst you deal with ringing the Microbiologist for advice. Medicine for the most part is all about being a team player, knowing your role within the team, and supporting others within it.

3. Demonstrate increasing ability to communicate with patients in more challenging circumstances and deal independently with queries from patients and relatives

As an F1 you are not technically supposed to do your own ward rounds (you can label them 'Ward Reviews' but you shouldn't be regularly doing rounds unsupervised). For an F2 this is all change. You now will often be expected to go round the wards with your junior and deal directly with the patients and any problems they throw up. You will have to become competent in breaking bad news, recognising when capacity is impaired and how to proceed, discuss-

ing DNAR orders, taking part in the referral process between primary and secondary care, recognising situations which might lead to a complaint (and engage in damage limitation), and often you will need to obtain consent (F1s are not allowed to fill in consent forms). With regards to consent, do remember it's illegal to obtain consent unless the patient (with capacity) is fully informed of the purpose of the procedure, the intended benefit, and the major risks (see Appendix 1). Only someone who is au fait with the ins and outs of the procedure should be the person obtaining consent. **If this isn't you then don't do it**! If, for example you are a Cardiology SHO, perhaps go along one afternoon to the Cath Lab to watch a few angiograms before getting folk to sign that yellow form, and make sure that your consultant and Trust policy is happy with you doing it. Don't blag these things. It's really not fair on the patients.

You will also have to have a lot of interface with 'angry rellies' and placate and reassure them. No matter how brilliant your hospital is, and no matter how hard you work, relatives might find their loved one's situation doesn't meet their expectations, and will 'want to talk to a doctor' in order to discuss their concerns. Remember Point 1. Be professional at all times. Don't let their emotions affect yours, especially if they are enraged. This will invariably make things *much* worse. Just stay calm, and more often than not, ventilating their concerns will make them feel much better. Try and work together to come up with solutions to the relatives' concerns, as this will make them satisfied that something is being done. The vast majority of these problems are down to a basic lack of communication between the doctors and the patient/patient's relatives. Try to learn from these experiences and honestly question whether you, or the team, could have done something differently.

4. Manages, analyses and presents at least one quality improvement project and uses the results to improve patient care

You know what they are talking about, don't you? Why, Audit of course! F1s could often escape under the radar with this one, but you must have at least one audit under your belt by the time you finish F2. Simple as. No excuses. Ideally, we should be doing at least one a year. Audits can be excruciatingly boring, I'm not gonna lie. There's a reason we all decided to buzz around in stethoscopes arm length in various bodily fluids and mayhem. And that was so we could avoid sitting in an office, staring at an Excel spreadsheet for the rest of our lives. Little did we know then, that we would be scratching our heads looking at pie charts after a 12-hour shift in A&E.

But it's a must, and for good reason too. Nothing in the NHS would ever improve unless we evaluated how we are doing, and came up with ways to improve our practice. And it kills a lot of birds with one stone. The selfish reasons of why audits are good are as follows.

It's necessary to have one in order to pass the year.

a. It looks very good on your CV.
b. Interviewers for speciality training will almost certainly ask you about audit and clinical governance.
c. You get lots of points on your specialty application. You get even more points if you re-audit the same thing (i.e. 'complete the audit cycle.')
d. You can present the audit. Not only can you use this for a mini-CEX on presentation skills, you can also tag this as a local/national/international presentation in your speciality application.

It really is a must. I found the best way forward was to try your best to audit an area you are actually interested in. My friend Pete audited 'How Many Pages in Patient's Notes Don't Have their Name Written on It' and it nearly killed the poor lad. I want to be a surgeon one day, and so audited incomplete excision margins in skin cancers. I found that much more interesting and enjoyable. In all three hospitals I have worked at so far, I have to applaud my consultants for always piping up with 'audit opportunities' for the juniors. They will often have done the hard part for you and picked a topic they want looking at. Take them up on their offer – it will make you look really good and be a real benefit to everyone.

5. Teaches and delivers presentations, participates in the assessment of others and reflects on feedback

Developing yourself in the role of 'Doctor as a Teacher' is really important, and should really start manifesting itself in F2 if not before. As you go up the ranks, more and more people will look to you for knowledge and guidance. Presentation skills are a must and you should try and do at least one per rotation in departmental teaching. Remember to get written feedback (there is also an option to get feedback electronically on your portfolio these days, which is handy). This is important for developing your teaching skills, but also gets you more points on an application and is proof for your portfolio! Also remember to seize the opportunity to get it signed off as a mini-CEX (or CBD if it's a case presentation.) For your portfolio, print off a handout of your slides, and remember your feedback. You get points on your application forms for teaching, and assessors like to thumb through your file to see what you've been up to. A few pretty slideshows in there will break up the monotony of their day.

6. Maintains e-portfolio, recognises personal learning needs and sets SMART goals (Specific, Measurable, Achievable, Realistic, Time Limited)

Yes, the dreaded e-portfolio lives on. A necessary pain in the bum to make sure we are all competent and safe. After that nightmare weekend you spent 'linking' everything at the end of June in F1 when you left it all to the last minute and realised the deadline was *tomorrow*, you are undoubtedly now a pro at navigating yourself around that glorious webpage. What I would say to you is this: spread the workload. You really don't want a repeat of that time you had to go in to work on your day off so that you could pester the Med Reg for a CBD. It's happened to us all, and it isn't nice. *Try* and be organised about things. As with the F1 chapter, you need the same amount of competencies completed. I tried to live by the mantra of 'do one thing every week' – be it a Personal Development Plan (PDP), reflective log, a link on the curriculum, or an assessment. By the end of the year, I had more or less 52 entries – way more than needed, and 5 minutes once a week is hardly back-breaking work. It's definitely worth 'playing the game'. With regards to the SMART goals, apply these to your PDP – use it as best you can to identify some good objectives with regards to what you want to get out of your rotations.

7. Is trained in Advanced Life Support and initiates resuscitation

These days some doctors complete their Advanced Life Support (ALS) certification by the end of F1, but for me, it had to be done by the end of F2. There are usually only a few courses in your area throughout the year, so book early and get your study leave application form in on time. You usually have a budget of around

£300 for study leave, but your ALS usually takes the biggest chunk of this.

ALS is quite a fun day out, though if you're like me and get your knickers in a twist, it can be quite a stress too. It's very helpful to have your certificate though and means you are a lot more confident in an arrest situation. Whereas the F1 is usually stuck ferrying blood gases back and forth, the F2 usually gets to be a little more hands on, and once you have your certificate, you should be able to hold the SHO crash bleep and play an important role.

As a side note about study leave, the amount you get depends on the hospital you work at. Make use of it if you can – do taster days in areas that take your fancy, or go off on courses. It all looks great on your CV and I wish I had embraced the opportunity when I had the chance.

As an F2 you can now apply for your MRCP if you want to be a Medic, and you may be in a better position to do MRCS if for some inexplicable reason you like surgery. *Don't* do it if you don't feel ready. It's not a requirement for core training, or for passing F2, though to be quite honest, it does look quite good on your application. From personal experience I recommend taking at least 5 days' study leave before your Part 1. I also thoroughly recommend a revision course. I did 'Concise MRCP' – an intensive weekend course based in Bournemouth, and would certainly not have passed without it. Also, the 'ole faithful' online bank questions are brilliant, and quite addictive. But everyone

has their own revision styles so do what works for you. Just don't feel pressured in to doing it when you don't feel ready. You have a good couple of years yet.

8. Maintains and improves skills in core procedures

You're an F2! Start to build up that skills repertoire! This is what the rest of this book is all about. Certain things on the e-portfolio are recommended for you to have a go at – though don't worry too much if you don't get to try. By now you should be learning lumbar punctures, nasogastric tubes, paracentesis and pleural taps. Jump on any opportunity to do chest drains, arterial lines, central lines, femoral lines etc. If you really must apply for surgery, get into theatres and start assisting. These skills will really help you out further down the line. Please bear in mind you will have junior staff starting who aren't as experienced and will not get that venflon in first time. Give them a hand, and try and supervise and teach as you go.

What happens next? Applications, interviews and alternatives

Not only have you got to juggle all the responsibilities outlined above, but you now need to seriously start thinking about what to do next. Otherwise you will quickly find yourself unemployed and without direction. This is quite hypocritical from a personal point of view. For me, I knew I wanted to do Core Medical Training, but I didn't know where. I couldn't make my mind up in time, so decided to take the year out of training. What followed was an excellent year of travelling the world interspersed with locuming in Cornwall and Portsmouth to keep the funds topped up. It was a fantastic year, and I engineered it so I was in the country for applications and interviews (having finally plumped for the East Midlands.) However I do understand this is a somewhat unorthodox movement into the next stage of training.

From my experience people generally speaking do the following post-F2:

a. Apply in December of F2, get a job, and go straight into core training
b. Do the above, but are unsuccessful in their application
c. Go to Australia and New Zealand, and earn a tonne of money out there
d. Take a year out to do a Masters
e. Take a year out to do nothing in particular (guilty)
f. Locum.

I will talk you through the above options as best I can.

(a) Applying in December of F2, getting a job, and going straight into core training

So you've made up your mind, you know what you want to do, and you know where you want to be. Well done!! Unfortunately this means that during your hectic F2 schedule, you need to work on your application, your portfolios, and your interview skills. You are contractually allowed to have the day of your interview off, but that's about it.

Your applications open in mid December. You have to get a login to the medical training recruitment webpage, and it's all quite self explanatory when you get there. A lot of the application is a load of gumpf to fill in about your personal details, right to work in the UK, ability to speak English, lack of criminal tendencies, etc. If, like me, you completed F2 before you applied, you will need to attach a scanned copy of your 5:2 Foundation Achievement of Competency Document to prove you don't need any further training beforehand. You also need to tell them about your qualifications – both postgraduate, and your BMBS/MBBS/MBChB etc. You also have to list *all* your F1/F2 experience, and any locum or overseas medical jobs you have held. You have to explain any gaps in your CV. Three referees are required, so get these confirmed early. You will have to ask them later on to provide references for you (when that is, is up to your deanery). Lastly you need to rank which deanery you would like to be interviewed at. For medicine, you provide them with 4 choices. You then sign off the declaration at the end and Bob's your uncle.

With regards to the other questions they ask you, it will naturally depend on the speciality, but for medicine:

• Additional achievements (i.e honours degree, prizes, awards, etc.)
• MRCP (i.e. have you done any of it yet?)

- Training courses attended (all that study leave shouldn't have gone to waste)
- Achievements outside medicine (I had to write 150 words on an outstanding achievement outside the field of medicine. For instance, I chose the fact that I am qualified in British Sign Language)
- Presentations
- Publications
- Teaching experience. For example, 'Give full details about the type of teaching, your personal contribution and details of any feedback obtained'
- Clinical audit. For example, 'Provide details of clinical audit giving titles and dates, outlining your contribution, what it showed, and whether it was presented and the audit cycle completed'. Commitment to speciality. For example, 'describe how you believe you meet the person specification for the programme you are applying for. Include the particular skills and attributes that make you suitable for a career in this speciality'.

Commitment to Speciality is a mind boggling one, and I went about it by detailing a difficult patient encounter, highlighting things I did particularly well. You can find out what exactly they mean by this on the MMC website – it differs for every job, but is quite clearly detailed. For example for Medicine, the candidate should display 'initiative, drive, interest in the speciality, commit to personal and professional development, self reflect, and attend teaching'. The best advice for filling in all these prose answers is to look at the details of the 'Person Specifications' available on the website and try to make sure that you show in your answer, evidence of being all of those things. Remember the person spec is the 'Marksheet' by which they will score you on, so tailor all your answers towards it!

As long as you are eligible for the job, the vast majority of candidates will then go on to be offered an interview (for Surgery, you may have more than one).

Interviews are mid January through to early February depending on what you are applying for. It's worth knowing that prospective GP trainees need to pass an entrance exam prior to the face-to-face interviews. These are usually best of five answers, and are partly of an ethical nature. Practice questions are available online.

If you are applying for an Academic Clinical Fellowship (ACF) position they usually interview earlier, before Christmas.

On interview day, arrive early, and well presented. With regards to dress code, I think it depends on where you are going. Having trained in laid-back, beachy Cornwall, I thought I looked extremely smart in my jumper and skirt combo. However when I pitched up in Nottingham I was the *only* candidate not in a suit. I would therefore recommend a suit, just to be on the safe side. Even if they make you look boxy and uncomfortable, like they do to me. Make use of the water and refreshments, or else you'll end up with a horrendously dry mouth which could be your undoing. And most of all:

relax! What's the worst that could happen…?

Some people pay to go on expensive interview courses to help hone your skills. If this makes you feel more prepared then go for it. Just think hard in advance about the kind of things they might ask you, and have an answer to hand. It's crucial to have certain answers prepared that you can go on to manipulate to fit any question they ask, for example treating a patient with a seizure could be tailored to fit a question on clinical skills, teamwork, leadership, a difficult situation etc. What you *don't want* is to be left umming and ahhing with an awkward silence. You are throwing away an opportunity, plus it feels as uncomfortable as hell! It's perfectly reasonable however, and in fact advisable to consciously pause before launching into your answer and give it a moment's thought. You can do this without it looking like you're struggling.

Interviews differ between specialities, from a more 'traditional' format to an OSCE-style clinical examination. Almost all are structured, so that the examiners will only be allowed to ask you set questions. This makes things very boring for them, but standardises the process and makes it fairer for you. It goes without saying that to do well in them, preparation is everything so make sure you are familiar with the format beforehand and practice, practice, practice! Here are some of the common types of 'stations' you may encounter.

Station 1: Portfolio

You will have to bring a portfolio along with you to the interviews. A good guide on what to put in it is on the MMC website, but essentially, it should have *everything* that you mentioned in your application, and a CV. Any teaching or audits you have written about should be in there. It is essentially your evidence. Deaneries are usually quite good at outlining exactly what they want from you – for example I had to have two files, one for 'eligibility' (e.g. my references, immunisations and certificates) and one for 'evidence'. The assessors usually have a little bit of time before you're called in to leaf through your file and think about things they'd like to ask you. Then you go in, have a swift round of handshakes, and the firing of questions begins! They asked me about audits, charity work and teaching, and also questions such as 'tell me about a difficult situation you had at work' and 'tell me about a time you demonstrated good leadership' – these are very common questions, have something prepared!

Station 2: Clinical scenario

This varies depending on what you have applied for. In ACCS, you will usually have a SimMan and a resus scenario to navigate. In Medicine, we had a small vignette, for example 'A 20-year-old girl is brought in collapsed. How do you proceed?' and then we had to talk through her management. In GP, you might get a role play with an actor. It all depends on what they want to see from you. What I would say in this station is *Just remember*

A, B, C, D, E. You really can't go wrong with this. Don't get flustered trying to impress. Just go through the basics and you'll get there in the end. The assessors want to see a cool head, safe practice, and logic, as well as evidence you have developed your diagnostic and management skills over the past two years.

Station 3: Communication and ethics
In GP interviews, my friends had to perform a role play with an actor, often with quite a difficult content. For example, one of my pals had to chat to an 'OT on the ward' who was concerned because his doctor girlfriend was getting inebriated all the time, and turning up to work drunk. The assessors are looking at how you communicate, and how you would prioritise and deal with the tricky situation. For medicine, we had to discuss a difficult case surrounding a DNAR decision for a young woman with terminal cancer who wanted full resuscitation. In Public Health you may instead be asked to give a short presentation (often with a whiteboard prop) about an epidemiological issue, such as obesity and how to tackle it. It's always a dilemma – that's the whole point – but just stay calm and just employ common sense if all else fails. If in doubt, say you'd speak to a senior!

And then that's it! You usually find out within a month if you've been successful or not. If you've applied for two different specialities, it's possible to 'hold' an offer for one job, whilst you wait to see if you have got the other. Remember to accept as soon as you have made up your mind though!

(b) Doing the above, but being unsuccessful in your application
If you didn't get a post, don't worry. Training posts these days are increasingly competitive and a huge number of people end up being unsuccessful in their applications. It's obviously difficult not to get upset and disheartened about the whole thing, and you will need a couple of days to let this sink in. But don't let it put you off. There is clearing, for one thing, and you are often put on a 'reserve list' if you scored well in the interviews. Many people who have applied, for example for ACCS and Medicine will decline their Medical post if they get an Anaesthetics job (or vice versa). This will bump you up the queue. If all else fails, try again next year. There are lots of non-training SHO posts and locum posts available for you. Use these as an extra experience, earn some good money, dust yourself off and try again next year.

(c) Going to Australia and New Zealand, and earning a tonne of money out there
A *huge* number of my friends took a post-F2 year out to go and work abroad, usually to Oz or NZ. These will not count towards any training scheme in the UK, but you can earn very good money indeed, experience a different culture, and come back looking bronzed and

smug. The Gold Coast in Eastern Australia is particularly popular with Brits, in fact their hospital there is swarming with ex-pats, and there is a good social scene. Experiences at work vary, according to my friends. Some SHOs are treated like Registrars, and some are treated like Phlebotomists. If you choose to apply, please remember to factor in that you might well have to come back to Britain for interviews that January, and sorting things out from afar can be tricky. Also, try and get visas etc. sorted out in good time. Aussie immigration is notoriously brutal, and several of my friends have had jobs delayed because of visa issues.

(d) Taking a year out to do a Masters
Several of my friends have done this, often supplementing their income with locums on the side.

(e) Taking a year out to do nothing in particular (guilty)
If you are taking a year out of training, I really do recommend a spot of travelling. I had to save up for 1.5 years to blow all my cash in 3 months but it was worth it. Do be warned, on your return to the hospital, you *will* feel rusty.

(f) Locum
Locuming is underrated. I did it for a few months and it was great. You earn twice as much as you would normally, you get experience working in other hospitals, and you have a flexibility and power over your shifts that you never otherwise get. Of course, there are downsides. Work is not guaranteed, and there's often no continuity in the care you provide. It can be confusing and isolating being in a new place every week with no computer access and no support! My advice is to join an agency, and aim for posts that are at least a couple of weeks long, or at least attempt to return to the same department. My locum job in Portsmouth was a couple of months long, plenty of time to learn the ropes and know the patients. Much better than it feeling like Black Wednesday every day!! Be aware though, some employers may see it as a negative if you have spent a year or so locuming as they may interpret it as you have not had career direction. Be prepared to justify it at interview.

Curriculum vitae
As detailed above, you will need to bring along an up-to-date CV to your interview day. If you are going abroad or locuming, it's also imperative to have a good one. At my Foundation Deanery, it was a requirement for my portfolio in order to be signed off for F2. So you'd best do it. Don't leave it until the last minute, and try and keep it updated every few weeks.

During shortlisting, it's unlikely that a potential employer would spend more than about 10–20 seconds looking at it so make it concise and to the point, with your 'big hitters' right up there at the start. It goes without saying that your CV should be an accurate reflection of your achievements. In short: don't make it up! At your interview you should be prepared to have evidence for everything you mention on your CV. Don't include anything that you don't have evidence for. If it is questioned and later found to be untrue it could be a serious probity issue.

Summary

From my experience, F2 was a thoroughly enjoyable year. The abject fear I felt as a new F1 had long eased, and firm friendships were long established. I felt very comfortable working in a hospital I knew, with friendly faces I was familiar with. Please do make the most of it, and good luck in your future careers! You'll do great!

Index

Note: page numbers in *italics* refer to figures, those in **bold** refer to tables and boxes

How to Perform Clinical Procedures, First Edition. Matthew Stephenson, Joshua Shur and John Black.
© 2013 John Wiley & Sons, Ltd. Published 2013 by John Wiley & Sons, Ltd.